Contact Dermatitis

Traditional and natural treatments plus preventing future attacks

Covers allergic, irritant and photo-contact dermatitis, causes and products to avoid

By Sophia Richards

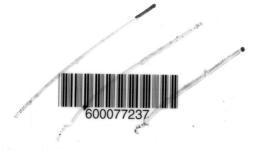

Table of contents

Acknowledgments

A huge thank you to everyone who helped make this book possible, with special thanks to Anthony, Dawn and our wonderful friends at the Primary Care Dermatology Society – www.PCDS.org.uk for their very generous gift of photographs within this book.

Introduction

Contact dermatitis is one of the most common skin ailments, and is becoming more common these days, as more and more chemicals are introduced to our daily lives. According to one study,

> *The prevalence of contact dermatitis in the general U.S. population has been variably estimated between 1.5% and 5.4%. Contact dermatitis is the third most common reason for patients to seek consultation with a dermatologist, accounting for 9.2 million visits in 2004. It also accounts for 95% of all reported occupational skin diseases. (Taylor J, Amado A 2014)*

Unfortunately, contact dermatitis is often misdiagnosed (usually self-diagnosed incorrectly) as sensitive skin or brushed off as "some kind of rash."

This is unfortunate, as contact dermatitis (both the irritant and allergen) can be treated and avoided quite easily, if you know what you're treating and what to avoid.

People who don't have problems with contact dermatitis might dismiss it as unimportant, but it can have an adverse effect on one's life, self-esteem and even work.

Contact dermatitis frequently occurs on the face, throat, hands, arms and other exposed areas, which can make the person suffering from it very self-conscious and unable to relax and enjoy themselves or even pursue a new relationship.

With severe cases of contact dermatitis, the incessant itching or burning can make day-to-day life uncomfortable and difficult to enjoy. The discomfort ranges from distracting to intolerable and it's often the inevitability of it that is most troublesome.

Contact dermatitis can even have an adverse effect on your work life and employability, especially if it is very visible. Contact dermatitis frequently occurs in people who work in hospitals, clinics, day care facilities and food service businesses. Unsightly rashes and lesions can cause customers or patients to become uncomfortable, leading employers to become uncomfortable as well, especially if they don't know or understand that substances in the workplace are actually to blame and that the condition is not at all contagious.

For all of these reasons, it's important to know if you have contact dermatitis, which type you do have, what has caused it and what you can do about it.

This book is intended to help answer those questions for you so that you can get back to enjoying your life and being comfortable in your own skin.

Chapter 1: What is Contact Dermatitis?

Contact dermatitis is one of the most common skin ailments. *Dermatitis* simply means inflammation of the skin and it's an immune response to the skin coming into contact with a substance that it doesn't like.

There are actually three main types of contact dermatitis. *Irritant contact dermatitis* is a reaction to a specific substance or chemical that only affects the immediate area of contact. *Allergic contact dermatitis* is an actual allergic reaction to a substance and the symptoms often spread out from the initial contact area. *Photo-contact dermatitis* is a type of irritant contact dermatitis, but symptoms only begin once the affected skin has been exposed to sunlight.

A Problem, But a Superficial One

Despite the havoc it can wreak in your life, contact dermatitis is not a systemic (body-wide) problem. Although in some cases it may spread over a wide area or several areas, contact dermatitis only affects the epidermis (the surface layer of your skin) and the outer dermis (the layer just beneath the surface).

This is probably small comfort when your face or hands are covered with red patches or you're plagued with itching and burning skin, but it is to your advantage when it comes to treating contact dermatitis, especially treating it yourself at home.

Contact Dermatitis versus Hives

Many people mistake contact dermatitis for hives or contact urticaria, but they are two very different things.

Contact urticaria usually manifests itself within just a few minutes of contact and often disappears almost as quickly or at least within a few hours. In general, contact urticaria is usually an allergic reaction, as well.

On the other hand, contact dermatitis is not always an allergic reaction. Irritant dermatitis is actually more common. Also, while symptoms may show up very quickly, they often takes days or even weeks to fade away. If you work with or use the substance that's causing it on a regular basis, they may not seem to ever go away. This is one of the main reasons that it's so important to identify the substance or substances that are causing your skin to react.

Common Symptoms of Contact Dermatitis

Symptoms depend on whether you're dealing with irritant contact dermatitis or allergic contact dermatitis.

In general, irritant dermatitis produces a more painful, burning sensation, while allergic dermatitis is usually just itchy. Both types usually appear as a red rash and some people may also develop hives (urticaria), welts or blisters. The rash and other symptoms usually appear quite quickly, but may linger for days or even weeks.

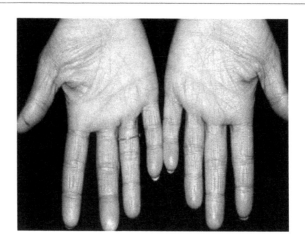

Irritant contact dermatitis, without the common rash.

(Image courtesy of PCDS.org.uk)

With irritant contact dermatitis, the rash is generally quite localized, only appearing in the immediate area of contact. Allergic dermatitis, on the other hand, can spread to different areas of the body, as it's an immune reaction to an actual allergen.

Photoallergic contact dermatitis, a subtype of contact dermatitis, has symptoms which may be harder to pin down. With this type of dermatitis, symptoms only appear when the affected skin is then exposed to sunlight or other types of UV light.

The Difficulties in Diagnosis and Differentiation

One of the problems with contact dermatitis is that people often don't understand the difference between being irritated by something and actually being allergic to it.

For instance, a cleaning product may cause a reaction because of your sensitivity to its harshness or alkalinity and this would be classified as irritant contact dermatitis. However, if your skin erupted because of an allergy to one of the specific chemicals in that cleaner, that would be classified as allergic contact dermatitis.

If you're fortunate, you may have an easy time figuring out what has caused your contact dermatitis. Perhaps the symptoms show up almost immediately after you come into contact with a new substance or chemical, or after a short time at a new job or hobby that involves products you've never used before.

More often, finding out what's causing your contact dermatitis will take a bit more work.

We'll touch on the topic of diagnosis in the next two chapters and in Chapter Four we'll go into more detail about how you and your doctor can get some answers.

Once you do know what's causing your contact dermatitis, it's fairly easy to treat, both at home and under a doctor's care. Avoiding the problem in the future may be quite easy as well, if you know exactly what has brought on the symptoms.

With any luck, the problem substance is one that isn't very common or at least not commonly used in your day to day life. If it is, well then you still have some steps you can take to protect yourself. There are natural alternatives to almost every household product or toiletry (and we'll give you some recipes for these later on) and you can protect your skin with either gear or a topical barrier. First and foremost, though, you need to know your enemy.

The good news is that once you do, you stand a very good chance of being able to avoid serious outbreaks in the future.

Chapter 2: Irritant Dermatitis

Have you ever worked in a place that required frequent contact with chemicals such as soaps or solvents? If so, your hands may have become raw and irritated, appearing as if they'd been burned. What you've experienced is irritant dermatitis, or ID.

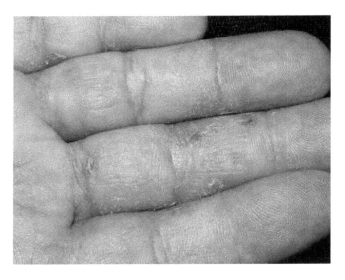

Irritant dermatitis, with cracked skin and reddened lesions.

(Image courtesy of PCDS.org.uk)

Irritant dermatitis is often incorrectly attributed to an allergic reaction to the chemicals. That's not the case, though. What's actually happening is that the chemical is causing physical damage directly to your skin cells. (Hogan D, Ellston D 2013)

Irritant dermatitis is the most common cause of skin disorders in the workplace because many professions require regular use of substances that can damage your skin.

Throughout the following paragraphs, we're going to discuss what irritant dermatitis is and what causes it. You may be surprised at some of the seemingly-innocent ingredients that are responsible for a good deal of discomfort to many people.

What is Irritant Dermatitis?

Irritant dermatitis looks like blisters or a rash and may make you feel as if your hands are on fire, or cause a constant, long-term itching. Because of its unsightly appearance, irritant dermatitis can be the source of a great deal of embarrassment in public. Fortunately, irritant dermatitis is one of the easiest forms of dermatitis to treat because it's the direct result of contact with a particular substance.

18

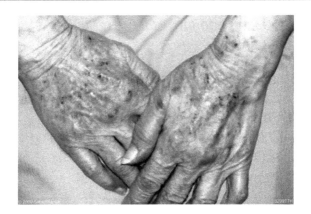

Widespread contact dermatitis on the hands, typical with a reaction to dish soap and cleaners.

(Image courtesy of PCDS.org.uk)

Irritant dermatitis occurs when you expose your skin to substances that cause damage to the skin cells faster than your body can repair them. Those irritants rob the skin's outer layers of their protective moisture barrier, allowing the chemical to penetrate the skin more deeply and inflict more damage. (Bourke J, Coulson I, English J 2001)

Though skin that is already suffering from other conditions such as eczema or psoriasis may be more sensitive to damage, healthy skin can be just as vulnerable to irritant dermatitis if it's exposed long enough, or if the chemical is powerful enough.

You may mistake irritant dermatitis for an allergic reaction, known as contact dermatitis, but it's a separate condition. Your skin is actually being damaged instead of reacting to an allergen. With irritant dermatitis, your immune system isn't involved.

We'll discuss allergic contact dermatitis in the next chapter because it's a horse of a completely different color, especially when it comes to treatment options.

What Are The Symptoms of Irritant Dermatitis?

This is where differentiating irritant dermatitis from other forms of dermatitis gets a bit tricky. Visually, it appears much like allergic contact dermatitis, though it tends to burn more than itch.

Typically, the symptoms of irritant dermatitis are limited to the immediate area that's come into contact with the irritant. Here are the most common symptoms:

- Red rash
- Blisters

_____

- Pain or sensation of burning
- Swelling
- Scaling or sloughing
- Glazed, "burned" appearance

The appearance of irritant dermatitis can vary dramatically based upon the irritant and how long you were exposed to it. Even excessive exposure to mild irritants such as hand soap can cause itching, dryness, scaling and cracking over a period of time.

Common Forms of Irritant Dermatitis

Though just about anything can irritate your skin under the right circumstances, there are several situations that frequently lead to irritant dermatitis.

Chemical Exposure

According to the National Institute of Health, irritant dermatitis is the most common type of contact dermatitis. It's commonly found in professions that require regular exposure to chemicals such as:

- Hair dyes
- Detergents
- Bodily fluids

- Shampoos or other hair chemicals
- Pesticides
- Cement
- Extended exposure to water
- Bleach
- Fiberglass

As you can imagine, the list of workplaces that involve exposure to these irritants is long. They include hair salons, cleaning businesses, restaurants, factories, pool services, hospitals, doctor's offices, construction sites, nursing homes, pest control companies and even agricultural operations. (Bourke J, Coulson I, English J 2001)

Diaper Rash

Also known as napkin dermatitis, diaper rash is exactly what it sounds like. It's a red, raised, painful rash that results from extended exposure to urine or feces. It's found in babies and in the elderly. Especially acidic urine (usually colored a deep yellow) is often to blame.

Dribble Rash

Since saliva is alkaline, it can irritate your skin and cause a rash or raw spots. Dribble rash is typically found in babies who drool or older kids and adults who lick their lips frequently. Since dampness is a breeding ground for bacteria, infection is a concern with dribble rash and may exacerbate the condition.

Winter Itch

Exposure to cold temperatures and the lack of humidity caused by running the heat in the winter can combine to cause winter itch. This condition can manifest itself anywhere on your body but is most common on your hands, face, feet and legs. Your skin will look dry and it may itch and get scaly.

Cosmetic Irritation

Cosmetic irritation is especially common in people with eczema and rosacea, for whom cosmetics can sometimes cause irritation upon application. Typically, the symptoms include burning and redness. Even after you wash the product off, you may still experience itching and dry skin because the damage has already been done.

Housewife's Eczema

Also known as dishpan hands, this condition is common among people who frequently have their hands in hot water, detergents, cleaners, and bleach. Symptoms include dry patches, itching, redness and cracking. This particular form of irritant dermatitis is common among people who work in laundry facilities, as janitors or housekeepers or whose work includes frequent bathing of patients or children.

Rubber Gloves

Though allergic reactions to latex or powder often account for irritation from gloves, it's also possible that the powder or traces of chemicals inside the gloves are just irritating your skin.

Friction

This may seem like basic common sense, but friction is a common cause of irritant dermatitis. Especially if your skin is wet, this can quickly cause open sores.

Now you know some of the most common causes of irritant dermatitis, but you also need to know how to know for sure what's causing your problems and, most importantly, how they can best be treated.

Diagnosing Irritant Dermatitis

The biggest problem with diagnosing irritant dermatitis is that there is no test for it. As you can tell from some of the examples listed above, the cause is often obvious and your doctor can treat it accordingly just based upon observation and your input as far as the things that you come into contact with frequently or have come into contact with recently.

However, there are often times when the cause of the irritation may not be so clear. In those cases, it's a matter of eliminating other potential causes such as allergic or contact dermatitis.

Differentiating Allergic Dermatitis and Irritant Dermatitis

Though it can be difficult to differentiate between the two, there are a few ways that allergic and irritant dermatitis may differ, including:

- **Location** – Irritant dermatitis will typically appear only at the site of contact. If you develop odd rashes in other places, it's most likely an allergic reaction.
- **Time** – Irritation usually occurs immediately following exposure whereas

an allergy may take as long as a couple of days to manifest itself or for the symptoms to become noticeable.

- **Painful or Itchy?** – Especially in the case of chemical irritants, irritant dermatitis tends to be more painful than it is itchy. Allergic reactions almost always include itching as a primary symptom.

Factors that can influence the severity of irritant dermatitis include:

- How long you were exposed to the irritant
- How strong the irritant is
- How much of the irritant you were exposed to
- How sensitive your skin is
- Environmental factors such as temperature and humidity

Treating Irritant Dermatitis- An Overview

Once you've determined what's causing your rash, it's easier to decide how to treat it. If the cause is obvious and the irritation isn't serious, you can often treat it at home. Here are some suggestions to help you get relief.

- **Rinse thoroughly** – Sometimes just flushing your skin with plenty of cool, clean water to remove the irritant will do the trick.

- **Moisturizing creams or emollients –** Use common sense here. If your skin is dry and scaly, moisturizers and emollients will help keep your skin moist so that it can heal properly. If you have open, oozing blisters, this isn't a viable option. Using a good moisturizer, especially one that contains barrier ingredients (like petroleum jelly) is an excellent way to *prevent* many forms of irritant dermatitis to begin with.

- **Avoiding Exposure –** Once you've figured out what is causing your irritant dermatitis, you can take steps to avoid the substance. Continued exposure will make your condition worse and may lead to infection.

- **Corticosteroids –** If the itching is unbearable, corticosteroid creams may be used temporarily to reduce the swelling and help with the itching. 1% corticosteroid ointments are available over the counter and are labeled as hydrocortisone. They help to relieve the inflammation that causes itching. However, you should speak with your doctor before using a corticosteroid cream, as prolonged use or use in the wrong areas can be harmful. (More on this in the next chapter)

- **Wet dressings –** If the damage is serious enough, you may need to use wet dressings to keep the wounded area moist while it heals. This also acts as an anti-inflammatory step and can help with itching and corticosteroid absorption.
- **Oral or topical antibiotics –** If your irritant dermatitis is severe enough, your doctor may prescribe antibiotics to fight secondary infections caused by bacteria that enter your broken skin.

If your irritant dermatitis doesn't get better within a couple of days of treating it at home, you need to see your doctor. He can evaluate your condition and help you develop a treatment plan that will expedite healing and minimize your risk of infection.

Irritant Dermatitis Prognosis

Irritant dermatitis can be painful and annoying, but at least it's relatively easy to treat. Once you figure out what's causing it, it's also easy to avoid.

Symptoms should begin to recede as soon as you've cleaned the area and the irritant is no longer in contact with your skin. Just like a bruise, scrape or cut, it should heal rapidly.

Prognosis is excellent, as long as you take care of the dermatitis so that it heals. After you've healed, be sure to take measures to avoid the irritant that caused the problem to begin with.

Finally, keep your skin moisturized and take particular care to avoid exposure to other harsh chemicals or possible irritants. Just taking these two steps will reduce your risk of developing irritant dermatitis exponentially.

Now that you know about the first type of contact dermatitis, let's move on to the next most common type of acute skin irritation: allergic dermatitis.

Chapter 3: Allergic Dermatitis

*Y*ou itch and your skin is red and irritated. No matter how much you scratch, it just doesn't stop. In fact, it tends to spread. Chances are good that you're experiencing an allergic reaction to something, also known as allergic dermatitis.

The most important thing to do right now is *stop scratching!* That's right; even though it may be next to impossible, you're only making the problem worse because you're damaging your skin even further. Scratching not only spreads the substance that's causing the reaction (if it's a surface irritant) but also prompts a stronger and stronger reaction from your immune system.

Throughout this chapter, we're going to talk about what allergic dermatitis is, what causes it and, perhaps most importantly, how you can treat it.

_____

What is Allergic Dermatitis?

Allergic dermatitis, also known as allergen contact dermatitis, is an immune response to an allergen that your skin has come into contact with. What, in particular, that may be depends entirely upon what your immune system responds to. In fact, an immune response is exactly what differentiates allergic dermatitis from its sister skin condition, irritant dermatitis, which we discussed in the previous chapter.

Since your immune system perceives the substance or material as an allergen, you may not experience the reaction immediately; it may take up to a couple of days. By then, there's a good chance that you won't have a clue what caused the reaction. Don't worry though. There are ways to find out what caused your allergic dermatitis so that you can treat it and avoid future recurrences.

What Are the Symptoms of Allergic Dermatitis?

Allergic dermatitis shares many of the same symptoms as irritant dermatitis though it tends to itch instead of burn. Symptoms include:

- Redness

- Rash, possibly streaky and/or patchy
- Welts
- Scaling or Sloughing
- Itching
- Inflammation
- Blisters
- Open sores or crusting

The symptoms of allergic dermatitis can vary largely and generally depend upon the irritant and your immune response.

In addition to the symptoms listed above, the affected area may feel warm to the touch.

Common Forms of Allergic Dermatitis

Though you can have an allergic reaction to nearly anything, there are some substances that are particularly notorious for causing widespread dermatological chaos. Some of them you've likely heard of but a few may surprise you.

Plants

If you've ever gone camping, you've probably heard of poison ivy, poison oak or poison sumac. Contact with any of these plants are almost sure to cause itchy, blistery rashes that spread and are even contagious.

The oils from the plant get onto your skin and cause a reaction within 12 hours or so. The itching can be nearly unbearable but refraining from doing so is imperative in order to avoid infection.

Methylisothiazolinone

You don't have to be able to pronounce it to be allergic to it. This is a preservative frequently found in baby wipes, face wipes and hair products. Once it comes into contact with your face, it can often cause a red, itchy, burning rash almost immediately. (Hogan D, Ellston D 2013)

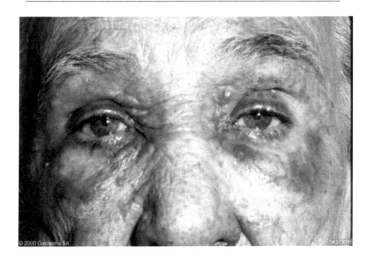

An example of allergic contact dermatitis contracted through eye cream.

(Image courtesy of PCDS.org.uk)

Rubber Gloves

Most people who have a reaction to rubber gloves believe that it's the latex that causes the problem, but that's not necessarily true. The reaction could be caused by a reaction to the powder or to accelerator chemicals that are used during the manufacturing process. Regardless of the reason, rubber gloves are taboo for a significant number of people. The problem here is that foregoing gloves may expose your skin to other substances that can cause either an allergic reaction or irritation.

Nickel Allergies

One of the most common fillers in jewelry is nickel. Many people are allergic to this, though the itchy red rash may be attributed incorrectly to the gold or silver that the jewelry also contains.

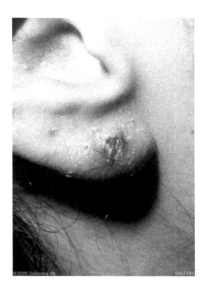

An example of reaction to nickel in earrings.

(Image courtesy of PCDS.org.uk)

Reactions to nickel may occur within minutes or hours of wearing the jewelry and are most common on the wrists or fingers.

Perfumes

We all love to smell good when we're leaving the house but a nasty red rash caused by your perfume is counterproductive to the pleasant appearance that you're trying to achieve. An allergy to perfumes and colognes is extremely common, though the allergy is actually to one of the chemicals in the scent, rather than the product itself.

Many people are allergic to ingredients in perfumes but there's good news. Though there are more than 5000 separate scents that are used in perfumes and colognes today, only a handful of them are known to be common allergens. As a matter of fact, there are only eight. They are:

- **Cinnamic alcohol –** smells like hyacinth. It's an ester found in natural scents such as Balsam of Peru and cinnamon leaves. Cinnamic alcohol is used in perfumes, deodorants, laundry soaps, chewing gum, toothpaste, mouthwash and some beverages.

- **Cinnamic aldehyde –** This has a warm, spicy scent and is found in cinnamon oil. It tastes like cinnamon.
- **Eugenol –** This has a strong clove scent and flavor and is found in clove oil, roses, hyacinths, violets, carnations and cinnamon leaves. It's used in everything from perfumes and hair cosmetics to aftershave, toothpaste, food products, insecticides and dental cements.
- **Isoeugenol –** This has a lighter clove scent and is found in essential oils such as ylang- ylang and nutmeg.
- **Geraniol –** This smells like a rose and makes up a significant portion of geranium oil, rose oil, lavender oil, citronella oil and jasmine oil. It's used mostly to make perfumes and to scent personal care products.
- **Alpha amyl cinnamic alcohol –** This has a strong jasmine scent and is found in synthetic essential oils. It's used in perfumes, toothpaste and to scent personal care items
- **Oak moss absolute –** This has an earthy, "oaky" scent and is an essential oil derived from tree moss. It's commonly used in men's products including aftershave and cologne.

Many perfumes do not come with ingredients lists, but if you do identify one of these chemicals as being your problem substance, your dermatologist or allergist has access to a database that lists all products known to contain that substance. This will make it easier for you to eliminate or avoid problem products.

Adhesives

Epoxy resins are used in a variety of different adhesives because of their resistance to many different chemicals and environments and because they're just tough in general. They're also a common source of contact dermatitis.

There are three ingredients in epoxy systems that are common allergens. They include:

- Epoxy resin, also known as bisphenol A
- Catalysts and curing agents that speed polymerization.
- Additives and diluents

This allergy is common among hobbyists, mechanics and home builders as well as with do-it-yourselfers.

Topical Medications

Just as you can be allergic to medications that you take orally, topical medications may also cause an allergic reaction. The most common medications that cause allergic dermatitis include:

- Neomycin, an antibiotic
- Corticosteroids
- Benzocaine, a topical anesthetic
- Salicylate – the main ingredient in aspirin that's often found in muscle pain creams
- NSAIDs – anti-inflammatories often found in muscle and joint creams

Photoallergy

There are some allergens that don't actually affect you unless they're exposed to sun. These include reactions to sunscreen, which is activated in the sun, and antibacterial soaps, which have ingredients that react chemically with sunlight.

Soaps

Perhaps the most common cause of allergic dermatitis is body soaps and laundry detergents. Though there are many different chemicals used in these, people react differently to each one and what affects you may not have any affect at all on your neighbor or even your kids.

Still, this is a huge category and we would be remiss if we left it out. If you have a reaction that covers your entire body, it could very well be your soap or your detergent.

Just as your skin is unique, so are your sensitivities so there's no way that we could compile a list that includes all possible allergens. As a matter of fact, something that you've used regularly for years can become an allergen overnight depending upon the whims of your immune system.

Allergic Dermatitis Prognosis

As long as you can figure out what's causing your allergic reaction, your prognosis is great. There are many different tests and procedures that you and your doctor can use to find the substances that are causing your irritation. Just remember not to change more than one thing at a time or you may never find out for sure what's causing it.

Chapter Four: Photoallergic Contact Dermatitis

This sub-type of contact dermatitis deserves its own section, primarily because it goes by so many names and has several sub-types of its own.

In the very simplest terms, photoallergic contact dermatitis occurs when the skin comes into contact with a substance and only becomes irritated when the affected skin is then exposed to UV rays. (Kerr A, Ferguson J 2010)

Photoallergic contact dermatitis can also be referred to as:

- Photosensitive contact dermatitis

- Photo-activated contact dermatitis

- Photocontact dermatitis

- Photo-activated contact dermatitis

The sheer number of terms applied to this particular type of contact dermatitis only serves to confuse those who have it and often lead them to information that doesn't actually apply to their condition. Here, we'll try to simplify things a bit to help you understand what photoallergic contact dermatitis (by any of its names) actually is.

What is Photoallergic Contact Dermatitis?

Although the term "allergic" may lead you to believe that this subtype is a form of allergic contact dermatitis, it can actually be classified as either irritant or allergic contact dermatitis, depending on the reaction. If the symptoms spread beyond the affected area or take more than a day to appear, the diagnosis is actually an allergic reaction or photoallergic contact dermatitis. If symptoms appear within a few hours of contact and remain local to the affected area, it's usually diagnosed as photo-contact or photosensitive irritant dermatitis.

One comprehensive study describes photoallergic contact dermatitis in this way:

"Photoallergic contact dermatitis (PCD) is a delayed-type hypersensitivity cutaneous reaction in response to a

photoantigen applied to the skin in subjects previously sensitized to the same substance. For the development of PCD, irradiation with ultraviolet (UV) radiations, usually UVA is required to create a complete antigen, and the culprit substance needs to be within the skin at the time of UVA exposure. The incidence of PCD in the general population is unknown and is considered uncommon." (Foti C1, Bonamonte D, Cassano N, Vena GA, Angelini G 2009)

What are the Symptoms of Photoallergic Contact Dermatitis?

The symptoms of photoallergic contact dermatitis are much the same as those of "regular" contact dermatitis, although there may be a significant delay between contact with the irritating substance and the appearance of symptoms. This is one of the things that can make diagnosis tricky, for both you and your doctor. If it's some time before your skin is exposed to UV rays, you may have a hard time pinpointing what is causing the problem.

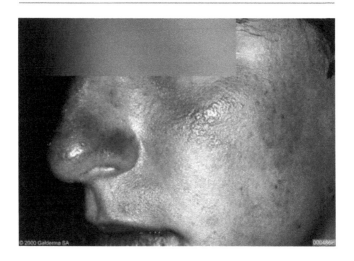

An example of photoallergic contact dermatitis.

(Image courtesy of PCDS.org.uk)

The following are some of the more common symptoms of photoallergic contact dermatitis:

- Red rash
- Blisters similar to those from sunburn
- Painful and often burning sensation
- Swelling of the affected area
- Scaly or peeling appearance
- Glazed, shiny skin as with a burn

One of the difficult things about photoallergic contact dermatitis is that because the eruption may happen hours or even days after contact with the problem substance but fairly quickly once exposed to the sun, many people believe that the sun (or UV light) is the culprit. If the symptoms don't appear very soon after exposure to the sun, the problem may be even harder to pinpoint correctly.

Common Causes of Photoallergic Contact Dermatitis

There are many chemicals and substances that can cause photoallergic contact dermatitis. The most common culprits are chemicals and compounds that are used to screen UV rays, such as in sunscreen and sunblock lotions.

Photoallergic contact dermatitis is becoming more prevalent today, because sunscreens are being used so widely. A recent journal article had this to say on the subject:

"Chemical ultraviolet (UV) filters have, over the last few decades, been increasingly used not only in conventional sunscreen products but also in many cosmetics and toiletries. Allergic contact dermatitis as well as photoallergic contact dermatitis reactions have been well documented as a

consequence of such use." (Hughes TM, Stone NM 2007)

Because so many of us are choosing to protect ourselves from the sun, these chemicals are being added to more and more products to make them more appealing to consumers. This is probably why we're seeing an increase in photoallergic contact dermatitis, even though it's still a fairly uncommon subtype.

There are several different chemicals associated with photoallergic contact dermatitis. However, in a recent study of 82 patients with photoallergic contact dermatitis (Rodríguez E1, Valbuena MC, Rey M, Porras de Quintana L 2006), these chemicals and compounds were identified as the most common:

Benzophenone-3 is commonly found in sunscreens, sunblocks and cosmetics that contain some amount of sun protection. It may also be listed on ingredients labels as oxybenzone or by its properties, 2-hydroxy-4-methoxybenzophenone.

Octyl-methoxycinnamate is also known as octinoxate and by the trade names Eusolex 2292 and Uvinul MC80. This natural compound may also be listed on ingredients labels by its properties, 2-enoic acid 2-ethylhexyl ester. It's one of the most common ingredients in sunscreen and sunblock. It's also commonly found in lip balms, especially those that are formulated to provide some sun protection.

Benzophenone-4 is also called sulisobenzone and is sometimes listed on labels by its properties, 4-Hydroxy-2-methoxy-5-(oxo-phenylmethyl) benzene sulfonic acid. Its primary function is to provide protection from UV rays, but it's found not only in sunscreen and sunblock but many cosmetics, shampoos and other toiletries. Benzophenone-4 has also come under scrutiny because of its estrogen-mimicking behaviors and the belief that it interferes with and disrupts the endocrine system.

Phenylbenzimidazole sulfonic acid must now be listed as ensulizole on US product labels but still goes by phenylbenzimidazole sulfonic acid in many other countries. This compound offers limited UVB ray protection and is most commonly found in sunscreen products with lower SPFs. It's also commonly used in sprays and lotions that are advertised as being lighter or less greasy.

Methylbenziliden camphor is also known as 4-Methylbenzylidene camphor (4-MBC) and the trade names Eusolex 6300 and Parsol 5000. It's been banned in the US but is still approved for use in Europe and Canada, typically in low-level sunscreens and cosmetics that include some sun screening ability. It's come under fire as another endocrine disruptor and some studies have shown that it leads to abnormal growths in uterine and other tissues.

Octyl dimethyl PABA, also known as Padimate O, is a UVB screening compound that came into use after PABA was banned in sunscreens. Its typically included only in sunscreens that offer low level (15 SPF or lower) protection and can also be found in cosmetics, shampoos, conditioners, hair sprays and skin lightening creams.

Although sunscreens and sunblocks and the above chemicals that are included in them are blamed for the majority of cases, photoallergic contact dermatitis can also be caused by chemicals (these and others) in other products, such as:

- Coal tar products (used in medicated shampoos, ointments and soaps)
- Anti-aging products

- After shave
- Shaving cream
- Hair spray
- Shampoo
- Conditioner
- Insecticides
- Disinfectants

There are also medications that can cause a photoallergic reaction when you're exposed to the sun. In particular, NSAIDS and some allergy medications are known to do this. However, this is generally considered to be a problem separate from contact dermatitis.

Diagnosing Photoallergic Contact Dermatitis

Diagnosing photoallergic contact dermatitis can be a bit tricky. There are two reasons for this: the symptoms may appear quite a long time after contact with the offending substance and if your doctor or allergist tests you for the chemicals you do suspect, the tests will come back negative if your skin isn't exposed to UV light during testing.

The most effective and accurate test for photoallergic contact dermatitis is a process called photo-patching or photopatch testing. Unfortunately, photopatch testing isn't used as widely as it should be. It's used more in Continental Europe than in the US, UK or Canada, but even in Europe only about thirty testing centers were found by researchers for a 2000 dermatological study. Of those centers, only two were testing more than fifty patients per year. (Gonsalo 2010)

The procedure combines dermatological patch testing for allergy with photodynamic testing. In short, suspected problem substances are applied to the skin in small patches and then treated with small amounts of UV light.

Unfortunately, there are a couple of reasons why you may have trouble finding a dermatologist who can do this for you.

One of those is that because photoallergic contact dermatitis is fairly uncommon, not many dermatologists are up-to-date on testing procedures or diagnosis. Secondly, there are few dermatologists or allergists that have the facilities for both allergy patch testing and UV irradiation.

The best case scenario is that you're able to make a link between contact with a problem substance and contact with the sun or UV rays and then locate a dermatologist or allergist who has the facilities to do photopatch testing for you.

Prognosis for Photoallergic Contact Dermatitis

The key to a happy prognosis with photoallergic contact dermatitis is being able to avoid the chemical causing it. That sounds overly simplistic, as this is the key with all types of contact dermatitis, but we say this because it's often easier to identify and avoid problem substances with the other forms of the disease. Another issue is that if one of the chemicals used in sunscreens is the culprit, you may have a much harder time finding a safe substitute than you would if your enemy were bathroom cleaner. It's fairly easy to make your own cleaners, but not so simple to make your own sun protection or find one that does not contain the problem ingredient.

If the problem is sunscreen, it may come down to choosing between protecting your skin from sun damage and protecting it from contact dermatitis. That's a very tough decision to make. This will depend mainly on which chemical in your sunscreen is causing your symptoms. There are sunscreen brands available that are PABA-free and also made without many of the other problem chemicals found in sun care products. Sunsense, a product from Australia, is just one, though you'll need to look up the ingredients list to make sure that it's right for you.

If your problem turns out to be one of the chemicals in shampoo or perfume, you'll have more options for alternative products and a much easier time avoiding eruptions.

Chapter 5: Diagnosing Contact Dermatitis

Your skin is itching or burning and you're covered with red rashes or welts. You know you have a problem, but what could have caused it? This is the question that you need to answer in order to treat your condition and to avoid it in the future.

If you have a general idea about what caused your dermatitis, it will be easier to treat. If you don't have any idea, though, you'll need to figure it out.

Self-Diagnosing Your Contact Dermatitis

First, you need to know that there is no real diagnostic test for irritant dermatitis. If your condition is being caused by something caustic, the only way to determine that is by eliminating allergens.

In a nutshell, if it's not an allergy or some other form of dermatitis, chances are good that it's irritant dermatitis. Of course, common sense is going to be of tremendous use too; if you just finished cleaning the toilets without using gloves and have irritated hands, the culprit is most likely the toilet cleaner.

Even if you have no idea what's causing your misery, you can begin to narrow down the list of possible suspects by taking a closer look at your symptoms.

- **Does the dermatitis itch or does it burn?** Allergic dermatitis typically itches whereas irritant dermatitis burns.

- **Is the dermatitis on your hands?** If so, there's a good probability that it's irritant dermatitis.

- **Is the dermatitis on your stomach, back or other area that isn't commonly in contact with chemicals?** If so, it's likely allergic dermatitis.

- **Do you have a rash or does the dermatitis look more like a burn?** Allergic dermatitis is usually a rash whereas irritant dermatitis frequently looks like a burn.

- **Does the dermatitis get better shortly after you wash the area?** Irritant dermatitis begins to heal as soon as you wash off the irritant. Allergic dermatitis doesn't. As a matter of fact, allergic dermatitis often doesn't even appear for up to 48 hours after contact with the allergen.

If you can't manage to diagnose your dermatitis by using these questions, there are other tests that your doctor can perform in order to figure out if you're experiencing allergic dermatitis.

Throughout the following paragraphs, we'll discuss those tests in detail.

Patch Testing

You've probably heard about allergy testing that includes pricking the skin with needles treated with small amounts of allergens. Don't worry though – that type of testing isn't particularly effective when trying to diagnose skin rashes. Instead, patch testing is used.

Patch testing, as the name implies, involves placing a patch infused with a range of allergens upon your back in order to test for a reaction.

There are baseline allergens that are used, such as the ones defined in the European Standard Series of Allergens or in the North American Standard Series of Allergens. If there are possible allergens that are specific to you, then those may be included as well.

How Does a Patch Test Work?

It's actually really simple. The hypoallergenic tape has several small chambers into which your doctor will put the allergen. The strength is specially formulated to be strong enough to elicit a reaction if you're allergic but not so strong that you have a reaction even if you're not allergic.

There is a test, called the T.R.U.E. test, that already has all of the allergens in it.

Regardless of which test you'll be using, the doctor will put the patch on your back and carefully label it with the allergen(s). You'll need to leave it on for up to 48 hours.

After that, your doctor will take it off and examine you immediately for the first sign of reaction. He'll also look at the spot at least once more, quite possibly 48 hours later. As we've already explained, it can take that long for an allergic reaction to occur.

Your doctor will record your reaction to each allergen like this:

- Negative

- Irritant reaction (IR) – burn-like reactions, pustules, or sweat rash

- Equivocal/uncertain (+/-) – pink area

- Weak positive (+) – slightly elevated pink area or red plaque

- Strong positive (++) – papulovesicles

- Extreme reaction (+++) - blisters, ulcers

There is a chance that you'll have a false positive or even react to all of the allergens. This is called angry back and is most common in people with highly active dermatitis. It's also possible that you'll have little to no reaction to a substance that typically irritates your skin.

The European Standard Series tests for the following:

- Potassium dichromate (Chrome)

- 4-Phenylenediamine base (Hair dye)

- Thiuram mix (Rubber antioxidant)

- Neomycin sulfate (Antibiotic)

- Cobalt chloride (Cobalt)

- Benzocaine (Benzocaine, an anesthetic)

- Nickel sulfate (nickel)

- Clioquinol (antibacterial)

- Parabens mix (parabens)

- N-Isopropyl-N-phenyl-4-phenylenediamine (rubber antioxidant, leather shoes)

- Lanolin alcohol (wool fat)

- Mercapto mix (rubber antioxidant)

- Epoxy resin (adhesive)

- Myroxylon pereirae resin (balsam of Peru)

- 4-tert-Butyphenol formaldehyde resin (adhesive)

- Mercaptobenzothiazole (rubber antioxidant)

- Formaldehyde (preservative)

- Fragrance mix (perfume and fragrances)

- Sesquiterpene lactone mix (daisies)

- Quaternium-15 (preservative)

- Primin (plant)

- Cl+Me-isothiazolinone (preservative)

- Budesonide (topical corticosteroid)

- Tixocortol pivalate (topical corticosteroid)

- Methyldibromo glutaronitrile (preservative that releases formaldehyde)

The North American Standard tests for substantially different substances. They include:

- DMDM Hydantoin (preservative that releases formaldehyde)

- Bacitracin (antibiotic)

- Mixed dialkyl thiourea (rubber antioxidant)

- Glutaraldehyde (preservative used for sterilization, embalming and leather tanning)

- Bronopol (preservative that releases formaldehyde)

- Fragrance mix (perfumes and fragrances)

- Propylene glycol (found in medications, foods and cosmetics)

- Benzophenone 3 (sunscreen)

- PCMX (preservative)

- Ethyleneurea, melamine formaldehyde mix (textile resin)

- Iodopropynyl butylcarbamate (preservative found in cooling fluids, cosmetics, pain and wood)

- Disperser Blue (textile dye)

- Ethyl acrylate (acrylic monomer used in adhesives and coatings)

- Glyceryl monothioglycolate (acid perming solution)

- Toluene sulfonamide formaldehyde resin (synthetic resin in lacquers and adhesives, including nail polish)

- Methyl methacrylate (methacrylic monomer found in plastics used to make dentures and artificial fingernails)

- Compositae mix (ragweed, arnica, feverfew, chamomile and yarrow)

- Dimethylol dihydroxyethyleneurea (textile resin)

- Cocamidopropylbetaine (detergent and surfactant)

- Triamcinolone acetonide (topical corticosteroid)

In comparison, the pre-loaded T.R.U.E. Test series only tests for six allergens. There are also site-specific and occupation-specific tests that can be used. The site-specific tests are for people who are only having symptoms on specific areas of the body. These include a foot series, a face series, etc.

Occupation-specific tests include a dental series, a hair dresser series, etc. Finally, there are patient-specific tests that have been developed for people who seem to be having reactions to specific items, such as shoes or cosmetics.

Patch tests are where your doctor will most likely begin his search to find what's causing your dermatitis. He may ask you to bring in personal materials such as your shampoo, cosmetics, laundry soap, etc., so that he can include those in the tests.

Finally, photo-patch testing may be conducted, too. We talked about this somewhat in the last chapter. This just involves placing two patches of each allergen on your back instead of one. When they're removed, one of the patch areas will be exposed to a small dose of UVA light to test for a reaction. The dose is too small to cause a photoreaction by itself. This type of patch testing will make it possible to diagnose photoallergic contact dermatitis, the type that only occurs when an affected area is exposed to the sun or other UV light.

If patch testing doesn't work, or if he suspects that there is more to your issue than a simple reaction, your doctor may conduct other testing, including a skin biopsy.

Skin Biopsy to Diagnose Your Contact Dermatitis

A skin biopsy is a great tool to use if your doctor is trying to exclude other skin conditions including psoriasis, tinea or even the skin cancer T-cell lymphoma.

Since many forms of dermatitis look similar, a biopsy is really the only way to know for sure in some cases. Especially if you have a history of skin cancer, a biopsy may be a good idea.

A skin biopsy isn't necessarily as awful as it sounds. As a matter of fact, it can typically be performed in your doctor's office during a standard visit.

There are a couple of different types of biopsies that are commonly used to diagnose contact dermatitis. Which one you'll get depends upon the location, type and size of your skin lesion.

Shave Biopsy

This is the least invasive type of biopsy. After applying anesthetic, your doctor will remove the outer layers of your skin using a small blade. It's so small that you won't need stitches.

Your doctor will apply some medicine to it to stop the bleeding and to keep it from getting infected. You'll leave with a small bandage on the spot.

Punch Biopsy

A punch biopsy is a bit more invasive but still isn't horrible. After numbing the spot, your doctor will use a small punch tool to remove a small, round piece of your skin. The piece will be about the size of a pencil eraser.

Your doctor will apply some medicine to stop the bleeding and then apply a bandage.

Though there are two more types of biopsies including excisional and incisional biopsies, you'll most likely undergo either a shave or punch biopsy to test your skin in an attempt to diagnose an allergen.

What to Tell Your Doctor

If you're going for a biopsy, you need to tell your doctor about a few things, such as:

- Any medications you're taking

- Any allergies you may have

- Any medical conditions, especially bleeding or clotting conditions

- If you are or think you are pregnant

You'll receive explicit instructions to follow before your biopsy. Be sure to follow them in order to ensure the truest results. You don't want to have to do this again!

If your biopsy results reveal that you don't have any of the other conditions, your doctor will most likely diagnose you with contact dermatitis. You can work together to figure out how to move forward.

Now that you know how contact dermatitis is diagnosed, let's talk a bit about treatment.

Chapter Six: Medical Treatments for Contact Dermatitis

*T*here are a number of treatment options for contact dermatitis, whether your problem is irritant contact dermatitis or allergic contact dermatitis.

Which options you'll use will depend on the type and severity of your problem, the options your doctor prefers and the options that sound best to you.

The best thing that you can do to help direct your treatment is to know and understand the options that are available.

Basically, treatment options can be divided into the categories of non-prescription or over-the-counter topical medications, prescription topical medications and oral medications. Of course, these are just the medical treatments; in the next chapter we'll discuss ways that you can treat your symptoms at home without medication.

Over-the-Counter Topical Medications

Over-the-counter topical medications (those applied directly to the skin) are frequently suggested by physicians.

The benefits of these products are that they're usually inexpensive, they're easy to get and keep on hand and you don't need a doctor's appointment to get more when you run out. Many people also feel more comfortable with non-prescription ointments than they do prescription creams or oral medications.

Of the topical medications available over-the-counter, various types and brands of corticosteroids are the most commonly recommended.

Hydrocortisone

Hydrocortisone cream is a very mild corticosteroid that is frequently used to treat allergic reactions and skin eruptions from contact with known allergens such as poison ivy. Primarily, hydrocortisone relieves itching (perhaps making it more useful for allergic contact dermatitis), swelling and redness.

Hydrocortisone is available under a variety of brand names, including Cortisone-10, Scalpicin,

Itch-X and many others. Typically, store brands contain the same concentration of hydrocortisone, so they're usually a perfectly fine alternative to the more expensive brand name products.

Hydrocortisone is not recommended for use on underarms or near the eyes and it's not known whether it can be passed into breast milk, so you shouldn't take it if you're nursing a child.

Emollients and Lotions

Your doctor will probably suggest that you use some sort of emollient or heavy-duty moisturizer on the affected area, to act as a barrier to the elements and possible irritants and to repair the skin's texture. You'll want to use a lotion or cream that has very few known allergens in its ingredients. Some of the creams most often recommended are Cetaphil, Eucerin, Aveeno, Vanicream and even plain old petroleum jelly.

Prescription Topical Treatments

If your symptoms are severe or don't respond as expected to over-the-counter creams, your doctor may ask you to take a prescription topical medication.

Topical Corticosteroid Cream

Prescription-strength corticosteroid cream is the most common choice among physicians for treatment of mild to moderate contact dermatitis, either allergic or irritant.

There are several different types or classes of corticosteroid creams available by prescription. Class 1 corticosteroid cream is usually advised for treatment of the skin of the hands, arms, trunk and legs. Class 6 or 7 corticosteroid cream is usually preferred for the face, as it's safer to use near the eyes.

Course of treatment

Treatment requires daily or twice-daily application for up to three weeks. The corticosteroid cream acts by reducing swelling and inflammation, alleviating itching and burning and reducing redness.

Possible Side-Effects

Corticosteroids can affect collagen production in the area on which it's being applied, which can cause a thinning of the skin. For this reason, it's not usually advised in areas where the skin is quite delicate or thin, such as on the eyelids or directly beneath the eyes.

Corticosteroid use has also been linked to glaucoma and cataracts when contact is made with the eyes inadvertently, so most doctors do not prescribe it for use near the eyes. If you have been prescribed a corticosteroid cream for use in other areas, you should not use it on a subsequent flare-up in the eye area without seeing your doctor first.

Topical Immunomodulators

In cases where corticosteroid cream has proven ineffective or when a topical treatment is needed for the eyelid area, physicians often prescribe a topical immunomodulator. Topical immunomodulators regulate the immune response of the skin in the areas in which they're applied (Khandpur 1, Sharma VK, Sumanth K 2004). One of the advantages of this course of treatment is that topical immunomodulators can be safely used for longer periods of time than can topical corticosteroids. Another advantage is that they are safer to use near the eyes, as some corticosteroids may cause a thinning of the skin, glaucoma or cataracts when used in the eye area.

Immunomodulators work by preventing the body's T-cells from producing cytokines, which cause inflammation in the affected area. (Lewis 2011)

There are two commonly prescribed types of topical immunomodulators being used today.

Elidel cream or pimecrolimus is one of the topical immunomodulators frequently prescribed for cases of contact dermatitis on the face (Katsarou A, Armenaka M, Vosynioti V, Lagogianni E, Kalogeromitros D, Katsambas A 2009) or for when the possible side effects of corticosteroids seem more probable.

Protopic 0.1% cream or tacrolimus is frequently prescribed for use on contact dermatitis of the hands. (Katsarou A, Makris M, Papagiannaki K, Lagogianni E, Tagka A, Kalogeromitros D 2012)

Course of treatment

Topical immunomodulators are typically applied at least once daily, usually for a period of up to two weeks. Tacrolimus is less readily absorbed by the skin and so can be used safely for up to six weeks if needed. However, this should only be done under a doctor's orders.

If symptoms haven't improved after two weeks of use, your doctor should be advised so that he can direct any continued use or change your treatment to something that may be more effective, such as an oral or systemic immunomodulator or corticosteroid. (We'll discuss systemic treatments in the next section)

Possible Side Effects

While, in some cases, your doctor may feel that a topical immunomodulator may be safer for you than a topical corticosteroid, topical immunomodulators are not without possible risk.

Pimecrolimus side effects are few and the common side-effects are generally mild. The most common of these is a burning sensation where the medication has been applied. This generally goes away within a few days, but if continues for a week or more, your doctor should be consulted.

Other common side effects include itching, irritation and redness.

Less commonly, some people may develop other skin problems, such as boils, warts, cold sores, impetigo (a bacterial infection), rash, swelling or a pins and needles sensation near the application site. If any of these occur, you should stop using the ointment and consult your doctor right away.

It's recommended that people using pimecrolimus not drink alcohol, as the combination of pimecrolimus, alcohol and sun exposure could put you at risk for developing skin cancer. (Lewis 2011)

Tacrolimus side effects are generally local and mild as well. The most common of these are itching, burning and redness. If these persist for more than a week, you should speak with your doctor.

As with pimecrolimus, you may also experience a pins and needles sensation, swelling or rash. These will likely resolve themselves, but you should consult your doctor if they last more than a week.

Other possible side effects are increased sensitivity to temperature, acne and cold sores.

Less commonly, some people may experience a swelling of the lymph glands due to infection. You should call your doctor right away if your lymph glands begin to feel swollen. It's likely not serious, but you may need a different course of treatment as well as antibiotics to kill the infection.

It's suggested that patients using tacrolimus refrain from drinking, as it's common for the combination to cause skin flushing and irritation.

You also should not use tacrolimus if you're allergic to the antibiotics azithromycin, erythromycin or clarithromycin. (Lewis 2011)

You need to tell your doctor if you are pregnant or breastfeeding, as tacrolimus is not recommended in these cases.

Systemic or Oral Prescription Treatments

In some cases, topical treatment may not be advised, usually if there is a potential problem with topical corticosteroids or if corticosteroid ointments haven't proven effective. In these cases, physicians frequently turn to systemic or oral medications. Of these, oral corticosteroids and systemic immunosuppressors are the most common.

Systemic or oral corticosteroids

Doctors often treat contact dermatitis with oral corticosteroids when the affected area is near the eyes, due to the risks we've listed in the previous section.

Systemic corticosteroids work in much the same way as topical treatment, except that they reduce inflammation system-wide or throughout the body. Oral corticosteroids are often used to treat disorders related to inflammation of the soft tissues, including asthma, arthritis and allergic reactions.

There are several oral corticosteroids on the market, but some of the more commonly prescribed corticosteroids are prednisone, prednisolone, methylprednisolone, hydrocortisone, dexamethasone and cortisone acetate.

Course of treatment

Generally, oral or systemic corticosteroids are taken for up to two weeks, usually once or twice per day.

Long-term use of oral corticosteroids can be quite dangerous, so it's generally advised that long term use be a last resort and only if significant patch-testing fails to pinpoint the offending substance and enable the patient to avoid the problem chemical(s). (Lewis 2011)

Possible Side Effects

Some of the more common and milder possible side effects associated with oral corticosteroids are nausea, dizziness, trouble sleeping, increased appetite and weight gain, muscle weakness and indigestion.

These side effects will usually go away once your body has adjusted to the medication, but if they persist for more than a week you should speak with your doctor.

There are some more critical side effects that should be reported to your doctor immediately. These include black or tarry stool, coughing or vomiting blood, swelling in your feet, ankles or face, prolonged fever or sore throat, significant weight gain, trouble with breathing, mood changes or any changes in your vision. (Corticosteroids - Oral 2005)

If you have liver or kidney problems, ulcers, high blood pressure, heart disease, osteoporosis, seizures, an underactive thyroid or a history of tuberculosis, you should not take oral corticosteroids, so be sure your doctor knows your complete medical history before prescribing an oral treatment.

Systemic Immunosuppressors

Systemic immunosuppressors are not commonly prescribed for the treatment of contact dermatitis, primarily because they suppress the entire immune system, rather than just reducing the inflammation response. This can be extremely detrimental to those at high risk of infection or to those who are already battling infection.

Usually, systemic immunosuppressors, such as Imuran, Neoral and CellCept, are only used when very severe, chronic allergic contact dermatitis makes it difficult for patients to work or go about their normal lives. (Hogan D, Ellston D 2013)

Because this course of treatment is far less common than the others, we won't go into great detail on their side effects and the course of treatment. If your doctor does recommend their use, please be sure to discuss with him any potential risks of infection (such as work in hospitals or day care facilities or a diagnosed immune disorder) before taking the medication.

Other Medical Treatments for Contact Dermatitis

If your contact dermatitis does not respond well to one or more of these common treatments, your doctor may prescribe one of these lesser-used courses of action.

Phototherapy

Phototherapy is sometimes used in cases of chronic and widespread allergic contact dermatitis, especially of the symptoms are not relieved by topical corticosteroids.

In phototherapy, psoralin, an oral photo-sensitizing agent, is taken and then the affected area is exposed to a very light dose of UVB (ultraviolet) light.

Common side effects of this type of therapy include redness, a slight burning sensation, skin sensitivity and increased sensitivity to sunlight.

Disulfiram

Disulfiram or Antabuse is an oral medication usually only prescribed to those who have a severe allergy to nickel. This allergy could be to the very small nickel content in some foods or to contact with the metal itself.

81

If nickel is found to be the problem causing your allergic contact dermatitis, your doctor will provide you with a list of foods and products where nickel is commonly found and may also provide you with a diet that excludes those foods.

Chapter Seven: Treating Your Contact Dermatitis at Home

Contact dermatitis is irritating, distracting, and sometimes painful and can have a very negative impact on your focus at work and your ability to enjoy your daily life. Happily, there are a number of things that you can do at home to help relieve the symptoms so that you can get back to doing the things that you need to do as well as the things you love to do.

Cold Compresses

Applying cold compresses can be very soothing, especially if your contact dermatitis symptoms include blistering. Apply a damp, cool washcloth to the affected area for a half an hour three times per day.

Coconut Oil

Natural coconut oil has been shown in studies to be highly effective in helping to treat contact dermatitis. Some people have used olive oil rather than coconut oil to help clear up their symptoms but unless you find you are specifically allergic to coconut oil, which is very unusual, it's going to be far more effective than olive oil and will give you some relief quickly. You can gently rub the oil into the affected area 2-4 times a day and it's worth doing just before you go to bed so your skin can absorb its benefits. You could also try adding a large tablespoon of the oil to juices and smoothies so that your body gets the benefits internally too. Try to purchase a high quality virgin and organic coconut oil for maximum benefits.

Aloe Vera gel

A high quality Aloe Vera gel, ideally pure or with very few other ingredients (or even the juice of a fresh plant if you can get one easily) can also be used to treat contact dermatitis at home. It should be used with caution however as there could be a slight chance that you could be allergic to Aloe Vera. Although it's quite rare to be allergic to this plant it is possible so try to do a small home patch test first by treating only a small area and waiting 12-24 hours to check the result. If it does feel soothing and doesn't cause any further reaction then it can be used 2-3 times a day to help relieve the symptoms.

Cool baths and oatmeal

Cool baths can be very effective at relieving the itching that often accompanies contact dermatitis. For best results, add about one cup of baking soda to a tub of water that is just tepid or slightly cool. You can also try adding finely ground oatmeal to your bath water. Aveeno and a few other companies make some just for the bath, or you can simply run the oatmeal from your pantry through the food processor until very fine.

You can do this as often as you like or as needed. Be sure to apply one of the emollients we mentioned earlier, or a natural product like coconut oil as soon as you've dried off, to replenish your skin's natural moisture and help reduce subsequent itching.

Calamine lotion

Simple calamine lotion can do a lot to help reduce itching, though it's more convenient to use when you're at home or when the affected area will be covered by your clothing. It may not be the best option on exposed skin if you're headed out to work.

Witch Hazel

Many people have reported relief with a pure witch hazel solution. Make sure that you get one that doesn't contain alcohol as this could irritate the skin. Again, it's best to start with a patch test by soaking a cotton wool ball with witch hazel and then dabbing a small area to see if it soothes you and helps reduce the symptoms.

Soft clothing

Wearing soft clothing may seem like an obvious choice, but it's one that's often overlooked. Even slightly rough linen, nylon, wool and polyester fabrics can irritate the skin by rubbing or by trapping too much moisture close to the skin and overheating covered areas.

Try to stick with soft, brushed cottons with a minimum of seams and detailing on the inside of the garment and in a weight and weave that allows your skin to breathe. Soft sweaters, lighter sweatshirts and sweatpants are also good choices. Avoid anything that is tight or that traps moisture in the areas where you're having problems. This might include bras, underpants, belts, sneakers or trainers, neckties, gloves, scarves, hats and pantyhose. Remember to wash and thoroughly rinse all new clothes before you wear them so that any chemical residues that could irritate the skin are removed.

Milk compresses

Milk compresses may sound like an odd idea, but whole milk is known to help relieve itching skin. Soak a clean washcloth or handkerchief in cool (not cold) whole milk and apply it to the itchy area for 15-30 minutes as needed.

Apple Cider Vinegar Solution

This has been reported by many patients to be very effective at relieving itchy contact dermatitis. Mix a 50/50 solution of purified or spring water and apple cider vinegar and apply to the affected area(s) with a soft washcloth. This is not recommended for use near the eyes, as it may cause burning and irritation.

Tea Tree and Chamomile Oils

Both of these oils have been used to treat contact dermatitis successfully. If you find that coconut oil is helping but you'd like to try an extra boost then either of these oils can be used – simply add 1-2 drops to your bottle of coconut oil - but again you need to try a patch test first to check they are not going to cause you more irritation. To do a patch test take a couple of

---

tablespoons of your coconut oil – add the smallest drop of whichever oil your testing and treat a very small area of your irritation. Wait 24 hours to check the results.

Any of these home remedies *can* be very helpful for relieving the itching that is so often a problem with contact dermatitis. It's best to try them in turn, starting with whichever sounds the most comforting, to find the one that works best for your specific issue. It's worth repeating that some of them, such as Aloe Vera and Tea Tree oil, should be used with caution, to check that they don't cause any further irritation. People sometimes assume that because something is a home or natural remedy then it will not cause any allergic reaction but of course this isn't always the case and it is possible to be allergic to some natural plants.

However, it would be extremely unlikely for anyone to be allergic to all of the alternatives suggested and you will find some that give you much-needed relief. Try combining these natural home remedies with the suggestions in the next two chapters, which can help you prevent future attacks and cure your contact dermatitis for good..

Chapter Eight: Living with Contact Dermatitis at Home and at Work

Living with contact dermatitis can be challenging, especially if you're not sure what's causing it. Not only do you have to deal with the itching, burning, and pain, you may also have to deal with social anxiety, feelings of self-consciousness and problems with working in a work environment that includes your chemical nemesis.

Throughout this chapter, we're going to discuss some tactics that you may employ to make life with contact dermatitis easier to avoid and easier to live with, both at home and at work.

Living with Contact Dermatitis at Home

Hopefully, you've been to the doctor and discovered which chemical (or chemicals) is causing your contact dermatitis. However, you may find your contact dermatitis has more than one or even two causes or that your skin is particularly sensitive to a number of substances.

Though the physical symptoms of contact dermatitis feel no better when you're sitting on your couch than they do when you're at work, at least at home you have complete control over every product that enters your abode, so managing your condition, or even finding out what's causing it, will be much easier. Being able to shed irritating clothes and plop into an oatmeal bath at will is also a benefit.

Still, avoiding irritants at home takes a bit of forethought and a bit of footwork; you're going to have to study every single ingredient label before you buy anything and also check everything you already have in your home to make sure it doesn't contain anything known to cause your contact dermatitis.

Check Every Ingredient Label

It will be much easier to find chemicals that won't burn you up or break you out if you know what you're reacting to, so please do get a diagnosis and allergy test from your doctor. Otherwise, identifying and removing problem products will be like searching for a needle in a haystack.

Once you do know which substances you need to avoid, you'll need to read every label in the house. This includes everything from bath soaps to toilet cleaners, so set aside some time to complete the job. Here are some products known to contain common irritants. You'll want to make sure you check all of these that products you have at home:

Perfumes

Dyes

Deodorants

Antibacterial products - often used to avoid infection from open sores caused by contact dermatitis, antibacterial agents such as bacitracin, neomycin and polymixin-B are actually known irritants for many people.

Hidden Nickel - Don't forget about zippers, snaps, buttons and belt buckles if you have a nickel allergy.

Rubber - don't forget about mouse pads, swim goggles, shoes, and even bra liners.

Alcohol

Retinoid products

Alpha-hydroxy acids, such as malic acid, lactic acid, and glycolic acid.

Sulphates, particularly sodium lauryl sulfate (SLS), is found in many soaps, toothpastes, and shampoos. It's a detergent used to get rid of grease and oil and also causes the soap to foam. Though not technically an allergen, it gets rid of the protective layer of oil on your skin and causes, or irritates, contact dermatitis by drying you out.

Coconut diethanolamide, a derivative of coconuts, irritates your skin much like SLS does. It's found in many barrier creams and protective hand foams. It may also be listed as ninol, witcamide, coconut oil acid, cocomide DEA, or calamide. Don't think that just because you can eat coconuts or even use coconut oil that this form of coconuts won't irritate you because it still may.

Lye – May be found in detergents, soaps, drain cleaners and dyes.

Latex – Check household gloves, bras and pantyhose. Interestingly, people with latex allergies also have cross-reactions to tropical fruits such as kiwis and bananas.

Ascorbic acid – this is used as a stabilizer and preservative in a number of products and is also the form of Vitamin C found in most vitamin supplements.

Parabens - look for these preservatives at the end of the ingredients list. Though sensitivities to them are relatively rare, they're present in many different products so you may be getting a lot more exposure to them than you realize. Also may be listed as parahydroxybenzoic. There are also tenuous links between breast cancer and parabens and though it's not definitive, many companies now offer paraben-free products in answer to public demand.

Balsam of Peru - This cinnamon-vanilla scented allergen is made of 60-70% cinnamein, a well-known allergen. The rest of it is made from various resins, which also may cause reactions. It's used as a fixative and as a flavoring or perfume. Rashes may present on your hands if you touch it or around your mouth if you eat it.

Preservatives - many allergy tests check for specific ingredients such as perfumes and chemicals but preservatives are also known to cause skin irritation. In other words, your lotion may get the OK from your dermatologist because you test negative to the "active" ingredients while the preservatives in the product make you itchy and scaly.

Formaldehyde - this preservative is used in many different types of fabric as a preservative. It's also found in trace amounts in food, too. Avoid it because it can cause, or irritate, your contact dermatitis.

A Word about Cosmetics

Cosmetics are a practically-endless source of irritants and allergens but there are several companies out there that make quality, organic products that are much less likely to irritate your contact dermatitis.

In general, look for products that have fewer than 10 ingredients, and make sure that you can pronounce and identify all of them. Your problem could be as simple as a bit of nickel hiding in your foundation. Here are a few tips to help you stay beautiful and rash-free:

Use PABA-free sunscreens, skin creams and foundations. Skipping the sunscreen altogether is irresponsible because of the risk of skin cancer but many sunscreens irritate, or even cause, contact dermatitis. Look for titanium dioxide or zinc oxide as the only sunscreens, unless you've already proven to be allergic to those.

Be careful with hair-removal products. These are often irritating so do a patch test first to see if you're sensitive. Same thing goes for hair dyes.

Don't assume that "unscented" means "fragrance-free" because it doesn't. It could just mean that the scent is masked by something else, or even that a fragrance is used to *make* it unscented by masking the chemical smell.

Unless you have an aversion to silicone, use silicone-based skin products. It keeps the product on top of your skin and may help decrease irritation.

Avoid water-proof cosmetics. You'll need to use harsher cleansers to remove them and that may irritate your skin.

If you develop a rash, stop using cosmetics on the area until it clears up. Though you may not want to walk around with a rash, putting makeup over it may, at the very least, continue causing irritation, and at worst, cause a nasty infection that will REALLY look bad and cause much bigger problems.

Keep it simple. As with cleaning agents, use products with less than 10 ingredients, and keep those ingredients simple. If you don't know what it is, research it before you slather it onto your face or body.

Use pencil eyeliners and eyebrow pencils. Liquid eyeliners often contain latex that can be a source of contact or irritant dermatitis.

Consider sticking with black eyeliners and mascaras. They are generally less allergenic or irritating than those that contain colorful dyes.

Use face powder rather than foundation. There are many good organic powders out there that will help to cover blemishes and give you a rosy glow without the chemicals and preservatives often found in foundations.

Earth-toned shadows are often less irritating than colorful ones. This may be attributed to the dyes and metals that are used to give the brighter colors their rich hues.

Replace your cosmetics every few months. They do expire and can also be a cesspool of infection-causing bacteria.

Do a patch test with new cosmetics before applying them all over. Each day for at least five days, dab a bit behind your ear in the evening and leave it on overnight. If you don't get a rash or irritation after that time, it should be fine for you to use. If you're particularly prone to sensitive facial skin, repeat the process on a cheekbone or near your temple for another five days just to be sure.

The world of cosmetics is tricky because many of the ingredients may sound "natural" but can still cause irritation. For example: Arsenic is a naturally-occurring mineral but you certainly don't want to use it to sweeten your tea!

The following list contains a few more general tips to help you keep your contact dermatitis under control at home. After all, that's where you spend the vast majority of your time, so it's only logical that you do what you can to keep it as safe as possible for your skin.

Avoid using bandages. Though you may be tempted to cover up your contact dermatitis with a bandage, the adhesive in the bandage may very well cause your irritation to worsen.

Change your air filters frequently. Dust mites are tiny, spider-like creatures that don't bite but

97

that are known allergens that can cause eczema. Change your air filters in your house every three months and keep carpets, drapes, rugs, and even ceiling fans free of dust because that's where they live. Also, they thrive in humid environments so keeping your humidity levels lower in your home may help.

Stick with cotton. Rough fabrics such as wool, polyester or synthetic blends may irritate your skin and make your contact dermatitis worse. Stick with natural, soft cotton for your clothing, bed and bath linens and fabric upholstery whenever possible. On the same note, buy shirts and underwear without tags or remove them completely to avoid irritation.

Double-rinse your clothes. Even if you're using detergents or fabric softeners with gentle or organic ingredients, they can still cause irritation. Many machines don't get all of the detergents out on the first rinse so double rinse just to be sure.

Don't assume that "organic" means "safe". Even natural products (citrus, poison ivy, cinnamon) can cause skin irritation. You can greatly reduce your risk of contact dermatitis by using organic products but you still need to be aware of what you're coming into contact with.

Don't assume that hypo-allergenic products are safe. This is a meaningless term used by many manufacturers to indicate that their products are gentle on your skin. There's no regulation of this term or any particular ingredients that are referred to. It's just a term and in no way implies that a product won't irritate your skin.

Wear powder-free gloves when cleaning and change them often. Sweating or getting water in the insides of your gloves can be just as irritating as touching the chemicals that you're trying to avoid. Change your gloves frequently to let your hands breathe.

Invest in a water filter for your sinks and showers. Unfiltered water, even city water, contains many different types of metals, minerals and chemicals that can cause irritation, dryness and allergic reactions. By filtering your water you can often stop contact dermatitis in its tracks.

Use soap sparingly. Because even the gentlest of soaps and detergents can irritate your skin, don't use them if you don't need to. When you do, stick with products that are tried and proven to be less likely to irritate your contact dermatitis. A few examples to try are

99

Dreft, Dove, Oiltum, Alpha Keri, Neutrogena, Purpose, Aveeno, Basis, Emulave, and Moisturel.

Watch your diet. If you have a nickel allergy, it's possible that you can cause or irritate your contact dermatitis just by eating trace amounts of it. Same goes with any food allergy that you may have. Nickel is found in varying amounts in fresh produce and meats, depending on the amount of nickel in the soil on which the food was raised. Your doctor can access data for your particular region, but small amounts can also be found in many packaged foods, making it difficult to eliminate all nickel from the diet.

Make your own perfumes, soaps, and hygiene products. We're going to share with you some fabulous recipes for these in Chapter 10 so you may want to give homemade products a try. There are several advantages to making your own products: you know exactly what's in them and you can make them exactly the way that you want them.

Keep your house cool. Heat aggravates contact dermatitis, as will high humidity. Of course, dry air can make dry skin even worse, so work toward a happy medium. Also, when you're outside, take what steps you can to keep from sweating because that can cause rashes to worsen. Also, sweat-dampened clothing can irritate your skin.

Rinse after taking a swim. Speaking of warm weather, chlorine and other chemicals in pool water can be extremely irritating to sensitive skin. Take a shower after you get out of the pool and apply a gentle moisturizer to avoid damage or irritation.

There are products on the market meant to provide a barrier for the skin to protect it from absorbing chlorine and other harsh chemicals in the pool. Skin Friendly's Nourish Pre-Swim Lotion and Joshua Tree's Watersports Salve are two you might want to try.

Keep Fido and Kitty clean and groomed. Pet dander is a common trigger for contact dermatitis. Buy your pet a nice bed to sleep on instead of sharing your bed with him and bath pets regularly to keep the dander down. Also, vacuum frequently. If you absolutely can't find another source of irritation, your pets may need to stay outside, weather permitting.

Avoid hot water. No matter how much you may enjoy a long, hot shower, hot water can exacerbate the symptoms of contact dermatitis.

Keep it warm but don't make the water so hot that it reddens your skin – a sure sign that the temperature is too high.

Paint your jewelry. If you have a skin-irritating piece of jewelry that you just can't live without, paint the surface that touches your skin with clear fingernail polish.

Just be sure that the nail product you're using is free of any known irritants for you. Butter London and Clinique both have lines that are meant to be safe for those with sensitivities to nail polish ingredients. As always, check the ingredients labels to be certain the polish is safe for *you* and as a minimum check that it is '3 Free' which means free from the 3 most harmful products traditionally used in nail polish (Dibutyl Phthalate, Toluene, and Formaldehyde).

Now that we've discussed some of the things you can do to keep your home as allergen-free as possible, here are some tips to help keep your contact dermatitis under control at work.

Keeping Your Skin Safe at Work

There are some professions that are more prone to high rates of contact dermatitis than others. If you've chosen one of these professions, you can still be perfectly happy, you'll just need to take some extra precautions to avoid itching, burning skin.

Some of the top professions for incidence of contact dermatitis are masonry, screen-printing, construction, painting, automotive, medical, dental plumbing, hair and beauty salons, restaurants, and healthcare/childcare positions. This is actually so common that there's a separate clinical name for it: occupational irritant contact dermatitis.

Symptoms don't necessarily all appear and it may take up to a few days for the symptoms to develop after you're exposed to the irritant. This is especially true if it's an abrasive or another substance that only causes irritation from extended or repeated exposure. Other irritants or allergens, such as acids, bases, or chemicals may cause a near-immediate reaction. There is, of course, also the risk of allergic contact dermatitis.

Whether your hands are exposed to abrasives that physically damage the skin or to chemicals that chemically damage them, working in these professions (and many others) means that you need to protect yourself a bit more than you usually would. Here are some tips to keep your skin safe as much as is possible.

Carry your own hand soap with you. Just put it in a small container and carry it with you in your purse or keep it in your workstation. That way, you don't have to worry about using questionable soap on your hands.

Change your gloves often. Yes, we've already talked about this under the home section but it bears repeating. Nitrile gloves are being used frequently in hospitals and other industries that regularly use them because of the many allergies to latex. It may very well be that you're not allergic to the latex but to the powder or to the powder when it's wet. Also, water degrades your skin quickly when you're exposed to it for long periods of time so changing them frequently is imperative.

Wear a protective mask and clothing when working with any known or probable allergens. Not only can chemicals damage your skin on contact, they can also cause dermatitis when you breathe them. Just like food allergies can cause skin rashes and itching, airborne allergens can do the same. Also, irritants such as fiberglass, sand, glass dust, metal dust or any other fine particles or airborne chemicals can irritate you from the inside out, or even cause damage upon contact with your skin.

Be aware of your environment. If you're downwind from a copse of trees or a field of flowers that you're allergic to, you can be in trouble. If you're outdoors, crop spraying with herbicides, pesticides or fertilizers are also something you need to watch out for, especially in largely agricultural areas. Also, if you're in area that has airborne allergens, such as an auto body paint shop or a hair salon, you can be exposed without knowing it if you don't make a point of being aware of what you're walking in to.

Wash your hands frequently. You're in constant contact with pathogens, chemicals, bacteria, and any number of other toxins, allergens, and irritants. Washing your hands frequently is a necessity but make sure that you use your own soap and rinse and dry your hands thoroughly after each wash.

Moisturize with a quality cream or lotion. Just as we discussed in the previous section, using a good moisturizer can help keep your hands from cracking and drying and may even prevent contact irritants from penetrating the skin as deeply should you accidentally encounter one.

Know what you're working with. Just like at home, be aware of what you're exposing your skin to. Check labels and look up ingredients that you are unfamiliar with.

Mix chemicals exactly as directed. Some chemicals are safe for your skin (or at least won't burn you in limited amounts) as long as you handle them exactly as directed.

Protect cuts or open areas on your skin. Nothing will make your contact dermatitis worse faster than continued contact with irritants. Cover them with a bandage or wear gloves but don't expose your skin to further damage. It just won't heal properly and you run the risk of infection.

Reduce Stress. Stress can worsen contact dermatitis so instead of skipping breaks to get that chart done or running down to get some coffee, take a few minutes to meditate and decompress. Also, avoid caffeine if you're sensitive to it because it can actually increase stress, which in turn will increase your itchy, scratchy, irritated skin.

Choose loose clothing and dress appropriately for the temperature of your workplace. Rough, tight clothing will make you miserable and if you're too hot, your contact dermatitis will be more prone to flare up and worsen. Also, heat makes the itching and burning worse. Dress comfortably in cotton, silk, linen or other soft fibers that won't irritate your skin.

Keep clean. As soon as you get home, take a shower to wash off any residual chemicals or irritants. Moisturize and take care of your skin.

Working in a profession that carries a high risk of causing or irritating your contact dermatitis can be tough. If need be, change professions but if you love what you do or quitting your job isn't an option, then you need to do what you can to make your job as safe as possible for you.

If possible, speak to your employer about using substitute products if a work-required product is making you break out. Of course, this is more easily done in some workplaces than in others, but see what modifications can be made to protect you.

Use common sense and apply the same principles to your workplace that you apply to your home.

Chapter Nine: Preventing Contact Dermatitis by Strengthening the Immune System

Contact dermatitis is an immune response to a chemical or substance that your body sees as a threat.

Many times, the substance responsible for that reaction isn't at all harmful in and of itself. For instance, the mango is one of the most nutritious and delicious fruits you can eat and the flesh itself rarely bothers anyone – yet, the oils in the skin of the mango are a very common cause for contact dermatitis.

The same is true of many of the chemicals and compounds found in manufactured products that have been identified as causes of contact dermatitis. Not all of them are necessarily bad. The products they're found in are also not "bad." But, for whatever reason, the immune systems of certain people just don't like them.

Our Immune Systems are Under Constant Assault

Boosting immunity is a hot topic these days. Health magazines, books, television programs and every other form of media are filled with information on immune-related disorders and conditions, the causes behind them and how and why we need to focus on healing and strengthening our immunity.

This is largely because there is so much in our environments that taxes our immune system.

There are environmental toxins and emissions, additives and chemicals in our food supply and substances in common everyday products that our bodies identify as invaders.

Overuse of prescription antibiotics reduces our bodies' own abilities to fight disease and infection by suppressing the immune system and disrupting the good bacteria in our digestive tracts.

Additionally, these antibiotics (and antibiotics fed to the livestock animals we eat) create resistance in the organisms they're meant to fight. In an ironically vicious cycle, our own immune systems have to work harder because we've helped various germs and parasites build immunity to antibiotics.

Our diets are not only full of unhealthy foods but lacking in many of the antioxidant-rich foods that we need to supply our immune systems with their "ammunition."

Finally, the pace at which we live also affects the functionality of our immune system. Overwork, stress and lack of sleep have a serious impact on our ability to fight off colds, viruses and infections because they create oxidative stress. That oxidative stress creates excess free radicals in our bodies; free radicals that our immune systems must fight.

Although there are few definitive studies saying that improving immunity will improve your prognosis with contact dermatitis, that connection only makes sense.

By doing all we can to help our immune systems fight against problem substances, we may be able to avoid or reduce the symptoms of that fight. At the very least, maximizing immune function can speed healing and reduce the time we have to deal with those symptoms.

There are two ways to boost your immunity: through nutrition and through lifestyle habits. We're going to cover both.

Boosting Your Immune System through Nutrition

Perhaps more than any other system in your body, your immune system relies on the foods you eat each day to provide it with the tools it needs to function properly.

Each vitamin, mineral and antioxidant has a specific use (often several of them) within your body. It's important to get a plentiful supply of each of them in order to ensure maximum health. Unfortunately, most of us don't get the variety or volume that we need. This is one reason why nutritional supplements are such a huge business today. However, supplements are not the ideal way to get these nutrients.

Why Nutritional Supplements are an Inferior Resource

Many well-meaning, health-conscious consumers spend a great deal of money on vitamins, minerals and antioxidant blends and other supplements in an effort to give their bodies the micronutrients they need. Many of us are religious in our habits of taking a multivitamin each day or drinking "health shakes" each day.

Unfortunately, these (often expensive) nutritional supplements are usually quite inferior in quality and effectiveness. There are a few reasons for this.

Inferior Ingredients:

Many supplement manufacturers cut financial corners by using substandard or synthetically-derived ingredients. This isn't true of all supplement companies, but it is true of quite a few of the larger manufacturers.

Processing:

Many of the ingredients used in commercial supplements have been degraded by the manufacturing process. Much of the processing involved in creating these supplements involve heat, which erodes the nutrient content much like the cooking process does with whole foods. Some nutrients are more sensitive to heat than others, which is why some vegetables and fruits are better for you raw than they are when cooked.

Age:

You probably already know that a carrot has the most nutrients immediately after being harvested from the ground. The longer it sits in storage and the further it must travel to the stores, the more nutrient content it loses. Then it sits in the produce section before sitting in your refrigerator for days or weeks. By the time you and your family eat this carrot, it may have lost the majority of its vitamin content.

The same is true of nutritional supplements. The ingredients used may be a year or two old before they're even shipped to the supplement manufacturer. They may sit even several more months before actually being processed. Once the supplements have been manufactured, they sit in storage before being shipped to stores, where they sit yet again. Lastly, they may sit on *your* shelf for months before being used up. During all of this time, the nutritional value continues to dwindle.

Insufficient Regulation:

While there are certainly manufacturers which strive to deliver high-quality products manufactured with integrity, the supplement industry itself is much more loosely regulated than you might believe.

Manufacturers are only required to list minimum dosages on their labels, even though the supplements may contain far more of a vitamin or mineral than is listed. This can lead to toxic levels of certain insoluble vitamins. (Jacobs D, Gross M, Tapsell L 2009)

Fillers:

Again, there are companies that strive to produce the highest-quality supplements as naturally and responsibly as possible, but they are in a minority. Most large commercial manufacturers are more focused on profitability.

Some of the companies known for manufacturing high-quality, less synthetic supplements are Arbonne in the US and Solgar and BioCare in the UK.

To that end, there are numerous fillers used in the production of supplements that never get mentioned on the ingredients lists. These include formaldehyde, carnauba wax, tar, petroleum, talc, isopropyl alcohols and even plastic.

Because supplements are not considered foods, manufacturers are not required to list every ingredient on the labels of your vitamins.

Numerous studies have shown that even a good-quality, fresh nutritional supplement is inferior in nutrition to the whole foods that contain those nutrients.

While a high-quality supplement is better than nothing ("nothing" being a poor diet), whole, healthful foods are far better than supplements.

Eating for Optimal Immune Health

There are a few different aspects to boosting immune health through nutrition. None of the body's systems are independent; each works in concert with other organs and systems.

This is especially true of the immune system, which relies on healthy liver and kidney function, as well as a healthy digestive tract in order to work properly.

This means that eating for immune health needs to include eating for a healthy liver, healthy kidneys and a healthy digestive tract. While that may sound like a tall order with a lot to remember, it really isn't. While our organs and systems are multi-taskers, so are the healthful foods we eat, many of which contain nutrients that support *all* of these important functions.

In this section, we'll look at the most important nutrients to eat for liver, kidney and digestive health and where to get those nutrients. We'll also discuss a wide range of antioxidants for overall immune health and which foods contain them in the highest concentrations.

Diet for a Healthy Liver and Kidneys

There are two sides to eating for a healthy liver and kidneys: feeding them the foods that are known to promote liver and kidney health and eliminating or limiting the ones that are known to impede it.

The liver is a hardworking organ. It breaks down and stores nutrients in the form of glucose, helps us to synthesize (digest and then use) proteins and fats and plays an important role in the production and distribution of several important hormones.

However, its primary task is to serve as something of a security patrol against toxins, allergens, pathogens and anything else that it perceives as a danger to our overall health.

All circulating blood and the nutrients and toxins in that blood must pass through the liver for processing.

When toxins, pathogens and other nasty items are detected by the liver, its Kupffer cells either break them down and convert them to something less harmful or send them out of the body via urine and feces. (Racanelli V, Rehermann B January 2006)

Limit Unhealthy Fats to Promote Liver Function

One of the things that can hamper this process is the ingestion of too much fat. The liver creates bile, which is what our bodies use to break down dietary fats. Too much fat, especially harder-to-digest trans- fats, means the liver has to devote time, energy and resources to creating more bile and digesting those fats. This is time, energy and resources that could be better spend on its role in immune function and hormone regulation.

Also, when these toxins are stored rather than eliminated, they result in excess free radicals in the bloodstream, causing oxidative stress, inflammation and slowed cell repair (including your skin cells). This is why your body needs an excellent supply of antioxidants (anti*oxidants* fight oxidation) such as Vitamin E, Vitamin C, folate, Vitamin B-12 and Vitamin B-6 in order to help your immune system work as it should.

To help cut down on the trans-fats and an excess of all fats, limit or eliminate fast food, deep-fried foods and high-fat processed snacks and meals.

Healthier fats, such as plant-based saturated and unsaturated fats and healthy saturated fats from fish, seafood, eggs, dairy and lean meats are much easier for the liver to digest and require less bile production. They also provide a number of antioxidants (Vitamin B-12) that further promote healthy liver function.

Eat a High Fiber Diet

Getting plenty of fiber, particularly plant fiber, is also an important key to improving liver health. Dietary fiber is needed to carry bile (and the fat and toxins it's carrying) through the digestive tract and out of the body. When we lack enough dietary fiber to do the job, that bile actually gets sent back to the liver. Essentially, it gets recycled and the fat and toxins are stored in fat cells around the liver.

119

This not only means that you're storing stuff better eliminated from the body, but that excess fatty tissue is being added to the area around your liver, which can lead to fatty liver disease and impaired liver function.

The best fiber sources are fresh vegetables and fruits, nuts and whole grains.

Get Plenty of Water

You also need to make sure that you're drinking adequate water. Your liver and kidneys need plenty of water for filtration and elimination process and your digestive system needs it as well to eliminate everything the liver sends its way. As a bonus, you'll also be providing much-needed hydration for your skin, which will aid in healing any outbreaks of contact dermatitis.

Nutrients for Liver and Kidney Health

All nutrient-dense foods, especially those rich in a variety of antioxidants, are going to help promote a healthy liver and optimal liver function. However, there are a number of specific micronutrients that are known to be especially useful to the liver.

Of these, **glutathione** is one of the most important.

120

Glutathione is made up of three important amino acids: glycine, glutamine and cysteine. What glutathione does is make the most of the antioxidants the liver has at its disposal by effectively recycling them.

What makes glutathione so important to the liver is its sulfur content. Sulfur is used by the body as something like a lint roller for toxins. Sulfur's attracts toxins to its sticky surface and carries them out of the body through your urine. (Scholz RW, Graham KS, Gumpricht , Reddy CC 1989)

Our bodies do produce some glutathione, but not nearly as much as most of us need, given the amount of environmental and other toxins we face each day.

Fortunately, we can also get and produce more glutathione from eating certain **sulfur-rich foods**. Alliums such as onions and garlic are highest in sulfur, but unpasteurized whey protein (made from dairy and sold as a meal replacement or protein shake powder) is also a good source. Avocadoes can help boost your glutathione level, as can the cruciferous vegetables, which are an excellent source of sulfur. These include cabbage, Brussels sprouts, collard greens, mustard greens, broccoli and kale.

121

Dark leafy greens are an important food group for healthy liver function. Their high chlorophyll content helps the liver to neutralize heavy metals and environmental toxins. Some of the best leafy greens are spinach, Swiss chard, turnip and beet greens and Romaine lettuce.

Sesamin, found in **sesame seeds**, has been shown to help protect the liver itself from oxidative damage. You can get it by eating the seeds or enjoying Tahini or sesame butter.

Citrus fruits, such as grapefruit, lemons, limes and oranges, contain phytochemicals that help your liver to produce bile, to not only break down the dietary fats you take in, but also break down and eliminate stored fats and the toxins in them. Citrus also contains important enzymes to convert those toxins to a water-soluble form so that they can be flushed out with your urine.

Catechins in **green tea** have been shown in numerous studies to support both the liver and the kidneys. These phytochemicals help fight oxidative damage to both organs, as well as elsewhere in the body.

Sea greens, such as **kelp and seaweed**, contain algin, which help absorb toxins and flush them out of your body. Their aid in neutralizing these toxins supports both the liver and the kidneys.

Beets are another food that supports a healthy liver. They're loaded with zinc, iron, potassium and magnesium, all of which are important nutrients for a healthy liver. They're also packed with fiber.

Turmeric is a popular spice used to flavor and color curries and other foods, but it's been used in Ayurvedic medicine for centuries because of its curcumin content. Curcumin is known to help protect our livers from toxic damage and can even aid in replacing already damaged liver cells. Turmeric also aids in bile production.

As we said earlier, some of the most important antioxidants for liver health are Vitamin C, Vitamin E, Vitamins B-6 and B-12 and folate. All of these are known to be especially important for healthy liver function. Fortunately, they're all very easy to find in everyday foods.

Some of the best sources of **Vitamin C** are spinach, broccoli, kale, kiwi, citrus fruits, papaya, bell peppers, strawberries, cauliflower and cantaloupe.

Spinach is also a good source of **Vitamin E**, as are sunflower seeds, almonds, Swiss chard, avocadoes, beet and turnip greens and shrimp.

Vitamin B-12 is found only in animal products and fortified grains. Sardines, salmon, cod, tuna, lamb and scallops have the highest concentration, but lean meats, organic dairy foods and organic, pasture-raised eggs are also good sources.

Vitamin B-6 can be sourced from both animal products and plant foods. Tuna, turkey, beef, chicken and salmon are all good animal sources. Sweet potatoes, sunflower seeds, spinach, bananas and potatoes are the plant foods with the most of this essential antioxidant.

Folate not only helps promote liver health, it also supports the regeneration and healing of cells, particularly your skin cells, making this an important nutrient for those with contact dermatitis, as it can speed healing. The foods highest in folate are legumes such as lentils, pinto beans, black beans, navy beans and kidney beans. Asparagus, spinach, broccoli and turnip greens are also good sources of folate.

Eating for a Healthy Digestive System

While these antioxidants and other nutrients are essential for the health of your kidneys and liver, those organs can't finish their job of eliminating toxins without the help of a healthy digestive system.

You also won't be able to absorb these antioxidants to begin with unless your digestive tract is functioning properly. While some micronutrients are absorbed from the mouth, the vast majority aren't available to the body until they reach the small intestine. There, tiny fingerlike projections called microvilli grab onto passing nutrients, absorb them into the bloodstream and send them throughout the body.

While plenty of clean water and foods rich in fiber are two of the main criteria for digestive health, there are other things you can eat and do to get your digestive system in top form and help your immune system to function more efficiently.

Glutamine-rich foods supply your body with one of the most important non-essential fatty acids for your body. We produce glutamine naturally, but if you're under stress or fighting off infection, disease or an inordinate amount of toxins, you may need to replenish your stores.

Glutamine aids digestive health (and your immune system) by helping your body move wastes and waste buildup through the digestive tract and out of the body. This elimination of built-up wastes then makes it possible for your microvilli to absorb more nutrients, including all of the antioxidants we're asking you to eat.

The best sources of glutamine are animal products such as fish, beef, chicken, pork, milk and dairy foods. You can also get a decent amount from beans, cabbage, parsley and spinach.

Recent studies have shown that the combination of **zinc and l-carnosine** can promote digestive health in several ways. First, it's been found that the two nutrients working together can help maintain the balance between good and bad bacteria in the gut. This is essential for a healthy digestive system and also has a significant impact on overall inflammation caused by an overworked immune system.

Second, this duo has been found to protect and repair the delicate stomach lining from the damages of oxidative stress.

L-carnosine is found in animal tissue and the best sources for it are poultry, beef, fish and pork. The best sources of zinc are beef, lamb, sesame seeds, pumpkin seeds and lentils.

Probiotics have become very popular in the last several years, as we learn more about the effects of stress and medications on our gut flora, the good bacteria that help fight off disease, infection and toxins.

Probiotics are basically colonies of living, beneficial bacteria. There are many different strains of beneficial bacteria, but most probiotics contain the bifidobacteria and lactobacillus genera.

The goal of using probiotics is to get these colonies to your digestive tract with most of them still living. Unfortunately, when you consume these bacteria through "probiotic" yogurts and other foods, most of them are destroyed by the digestive fluids of the stomach. This is why so many millions of bacteria are included in probiotics and it's also why this is one instance when a supplement may be better than a whole food source.

Of course, not all probiotic supplements are equally effective. It's important that your probiotic supplement be coated, to protect the bacteria as they pass through the stomach.

It's important to state here that most people don't need a probiotic on a regular basis. It's most likely to be beneficial if you've recently had an infection or have just taken a round of antibiotics, as both of these will kill good bacteria. Do talk to your doctor before deciding on a course of probiotics.

Getting a Wide Variety of Antioxidants for Your Immune System

While it's a good idea to target these nutrients that are especially good for your liver, kidneys and digestive systems, your immune system needs a huge variety of antioxidants in order to function at its best.

The best way to ensure that you're feeding your immune system properly is to eat a wide variety of plant-based foods, including fruits, vegetables, legumes, nuts, seeds and grains.

You've probably heard about "eating the rainbow." This phrase refers to the fact that different antioxidants are found in the various color groups of fruits and vegetables.

Beta-carotene, which our bodies convert into Vitamin A, is found in orange produce, such as carrots, sweet potatoes and winter squash. Lycopene, a powerful cancer-fighter, is found in red foods such as red bell peppers and tomatoes. Beets, Concord grapes and purple plums are rich in resveratrol, which is one of the most important nutritional weapons against free radicals.

The point is that by eating a wide variety of foods from all of the color groups (red, purple, orange, yellow and green), you stand a very good chance of getting both the variety and the volume of antioxidants that your body needs.

Lifestyle Habits that Support a Strong Immune System

While the foods you eat have a great deal to do with boosting your immune health, your lifestyle also has a serious impact. Many of our choices, habits and circumstances tax the immune system as much as environment and illness do. They do this by creating oxidative stress, which then results in an excess of free radicals roaming through your body.

Aside from eating a diet rich in antioxidants, vitamins and minerals, there are several things you can do to improve the function of your immune system.

Get Plenty of Regular Sleep

Numerous recent studies have shown that a lack of sleep, even in small doses, has a serious impact on our immune systems.

It was previously thought that this was true mainly because of the stress (and resulting free radicals) caused by lack of sleep. But new studies show that a lack of sleep can actually affect our bodies on a genetic level.

In one study, it was found that sleep deprivation for just one week increased the production of B-cells in the body. B-cells produce antigens in response to allergens and other stimuli. The researchers who conducted this study later found that long-term sleep deprivation had lasting effects that could lead to inflammation-related illnesses such as heart disease and Type 2 diabetes. (Vilma A, et al n.d.)

Try to get at least seven hours of sleep at roughly the same time every day. While this is a tough thing to accomplish in our increasingly overscheduled lives, it is possible. Record late night TV programs, set a time limit for doing work you've brought home and do anything else necessary to make sure you can get a good night's sleep on a regular basis.

Get Regular Exercise

Research into the direct connection between exercise and immune health is inconclusive and ongoing. However, we do know a few things about the connection between exercise and a healthy immune system.

By increasing the heart rate and blood flow, moderate exercise increases the speed at which white blood cells are distributed throughout your body. This allows them to be sent to troubled areas more rapidly, but it may also help them to identify problems much more quickly. It's also thought that this may also allow certain hormones to send signals to immune cells, warning them about detected bacteria and other pathogens.

We also know that regular moderate exercise does indirectly aid immune health by reducing

131

stress. Exercise stimulates the release of feel-good hormones, called endorphins, which not only give you a sense of wellbeing, but reduce the effects (including oxidation) of stress on the body.

It used to be thought that only extremely strenuous or prolonged exercise stimulated the release of endorphins. However, more recent research shows that moderate exercise such as walking, swimming or even dancing will result in the release of endorphins.

Reduce Stress and You Reduce Stress on Your Immune System

If you've ever noticed that you tend to catch a cold or flu when you're overworked and overstressed, you've glimpsed the very strong connection between stress and immune health.

Among other things, stress stimulates the release of cortisol into the bloodstream. Cortisol has several responses to stress, but one of them is the suppression of "non-essential" cells, such as B-cells and T-cells (the white blood cells) that our bodies use to fight infection.

When excess stress stimulates the release of too much cortisol, the number of white blood cells is dramatically reduced and you're less able to fight viruses and other illnesses. This is especially important if your stress level is consistently high.

You don't need to suffer the death of a loved one or go through a divorce in order to have a high level of stress. Job responsibilities, busy schedules, caring for your children and even a traffic-congested commute every day can do the trick.

Take a few minutes to sit down and list everything you can think of that causes you stress on a regular basis. Your list might include everything from a bothersome coworker to chaotic weekday mornings or the fact that you're never caught up on your laundry.

Next, try to write down one step you can take to reduce or even eliminate these stressors. Granted, some things may be out of your control (like your officemate) but you'll likely find that you can have some influence on most of your daily stressors.

Once you have at least one step to take to reduce each stressor (that you can influence), choose one or two of them a week to work on. Don't add more stress by trying to tackle all of your stressors or even all of the steps you listed for each stressor. Take it one step at a time and enjoy the impact that even a small change can make.

Even if all you do is round up the children's homework and backpacks before you go to bed, that ten minutes of aggravation you save in the morning will go a long way toward reducing your stress level and freeing up your immune system to tackle other tasks.

Boosting your immune system is not an overnight job, but it's not an especially difficult one. By taking a few steps at a time nutritionally and a few steps as far as your lifestyle and habits, you can make a great deal of difference without exerting much effort.

Not only will you be helping your body to respond more efficiently to the causes of your contact dermatitis, you'll also be improving your energy level, your mood and your looks with the changes you make.

Chapter Ten: Making Your Home a Safer Place for Your Skin

You've had your contact dermatitis properly diagnosed. You've identified the cause or causes. You've hopefully been able identify products that brought you into contact with that substance and taken some steps to try to avoid it in the future. Hopefully, you're also taking steps to boost the efficiency of your immune system, to speed healing and possibly even reduce symptoms in the future.

With any luck, you're able to easily avoid the product that has caused your problem because it isn't something you need to use regularly or because you've been able to find alternative versions that work just as well without the problem ingredient.

However, sometimes this is easier said than done. If your problem is an ingredient that's used in most shampoos or most household cleaners, it can be difficult to find one that you can use safely.

But, even if you haven't found a good alternative product, you may still be able to avoid future problems by making your own, safer version.

Safe, homemade toiletries, cleaners and other products are immensely popular these days, as people seek to make their home environments safer and more eco-friendly. There are numerous recipes available for making everything from glass cleaner to hair conditioner.

Sometimes, making your own product is just simpler, less time consuming and less expensive than trying to find a commercially-produced version that's safe for you to use without worrying about another bout of contact dermatitis.

In this section, you'll find some of the best versions of these homemade products, chosen for their easy-to-find ingredients, simplicity, effectiveness and kindness to the budget.

Pure castile soap figures largely in this section, as it's safely used by most anyone, even those with sensitivities to other soaps. It's available in bar or liquid form under several brand names, but Dr. Bronner's and Mrs. Meyers seem to be the most popular and are readily available from sites like Amazon and Ebay.

Homemade Household Cleaners

Household cleaners such as glass cleaner, dish soap, bathroom cleaner, laundry detergent and others are one of the most problematic categories of products for people with contact dermatitis. So many of the common causes for contact dermatitis are found in not just one, but several, household products.

Hopefully, one of these recipes will be just what you need to get your cleaning done without wearing body armor or suffering through a breakout of contact dermatitis.

Homemade Laundry Detergents

Simple Laundry Powder in the Blender

This recipe is extremely simple and economical to make and you can whip up a quart of this powder in your blender. You may need to work in batches if your blender is small or not especially powerful, but you can still have this ready in about ten minutes. Note that this detergent does not create a great deal of suds, but it works just as well as commercial laundry detergents.

Ingredients:

> 1 bar of Fels Naptha or plain Castile soap
> 1 cup washing soda
> 1 cup Borax

Instructions:

Grate the bar soap with a cheese grater, on the finest side that you can use comfortably. Grate the soap directly into a large bowl or plastic container.

Add the cup of washing soda and blend on low speed in your blender (in batches, if needed) until it's the consistency of a fairly fine powder.

Place back into the plastic container, add the cup of Borax and stir well with a plastic or wooden spoon.

Pour all into a smaller plastic container with a lid or into a quart-sized glass jar.

To use, add 1 tablespoon to the washing machine, just as you would regular detergent. This recipe makes 1 quart.

Simple Liquid Laundry Detergent

If you prefer a liquid laundry detergent, this one should do very well for you. This makes almost five gallons, so make sure you have a 5-gallon bucket with lid at your disposal.

Ingredients:

1 bar pure Castile soap
1 cup Borax
1 cup washing soda

Instructions:

Place a large saucepan with 2 ½ quarts of hot water over medium heat.

Grate the bar soap as finely as possible with a cheese grater and pour it into the saucepan of water once it's reached a simmer. Let simmer, stirring occasionally, until all of the soap has melted. Remove from heat and set aside.

Pour the cup of Borax and cup of washing soda into the five-gallon bucket and add 4.5 gallons of very hot tap water. Stir with a paint stick or large spoon until all of the washing soda and Borax are dissolved.

Pour in the soap mixture and stir again until everything is well combined.

You can wait for the mixture to cool and then decant into gallon jugs or just leave it in the large bucket with a tightly-fitting lid.

To use, add ½ cup for regular loads and 1 cup for large loads or especially soiled laundry.

No-Grate Liquid Laundry Detergent

This recipe is a great one if you don't like the task of grating your bar soap and cooking it on the stove. It is quicker and easier, but only you can only use this one if the ingredient causing your contact dermatitis isn't one of the ingredients used in the dish soap.

Ingredients:

> 3 Tablespoons Borax
> 3 Tablespoons Washing Soda
> 2 Tablespoons Dawn Dish soap

Instructions:

Pour the ingredients into a clean, one gallon jug. Using a funnel, carefully add four cups of boiling water. Swirl the jug carefully to mix the ingredients, and then add enough cold water to fill the jug to the top.

To use, add ½ cup of the detergent to each load of laundry.

Homemade Fabric Softeners

Fabric softeners actually add little to your laundry other than an extra layer of scent which may have come to signify "clean" to you. Many people who've had trouble with the ingredients in fabric softener report that they noticed very little difference in the softness of their clothes after giving up fabric softener. You may want to try going without it altogether, but if that idea doesn't appeal to you, here are some natural versions to try.

Nature's Easiest Fabric Softener

One of the best things you can use as a homemade fabric softener is plain vinegar. Vinegar is antimicrobial, a natural reducer of static cling and makes laundry wonderfully soft. Just use ½ cup of vinegar (white vinegar leaves less of a vinegar odor) in place of your regular fabric softener.

Homemade Dual-Purpose Softener

This recipe isn't as much of a cost-saver as
some others because it uses hair conditioner,
however even the cheapest conditioner will
work, as long as it doesn't contain any of your
problem ingredients.

Ingredients:

> 6 cups water
> 3 cups white vinegar
> 2 cups hair conditioner

Instructions:

Mix the water, vinegar, and hair conditioner in a
one- gallon bucket or container. Stir gently to
mix.

(Do not shake it; it will cause quite a bit of
foaming.)

Pour into clean spray bottles and spray onto a
clean washcloth to use as you would fabric
sheets.

If you'd like to use it as a liquid fabric softener,
store in the gallon container and use 1/3-1/2 cup
per wash load.

Scented Vinegar Fabric Softener

Pure essential oils can be a great way to enjoy a light scent in your clean laundry without the chemicals that are causing you contact dermatitis. Just be sure to select an oil that is safe for you and be sure that it's pure essential oil, not a synthetic blend.

Ingredients:

> One gallon white vinegar
> 30 drops of essential oil (try lemon verbena, lavender or any other scent you like)

Instructions:

Pour the vinegar into a large bucket or container and add the essential oil. Stir with a wooden spoon until well-blended and then pour back into the vinegar bottle and label.

To use, add about 1/3-1/2 cup per wash load.

Homemade Cleaners

Homemade Scrubbing Cleanser

This works beautifully on countertops, bathroom fixtures, chrome and stainless steel.

Ingredients:

1 cup baking soda

¼ - ½ cup liquid castile soap

In a small bowl or jar, add just enough castile soap to the baking soda to create a soft paste. You can add more if you'd like a liquid consistency.

Store in an airtight jar (such as a canning jar) or in a repurposed plastic container.

Natural Disinfectant Spray

Tea tree oil is a natural disinfectant and has a pleasant, fresh scent. This is great for cleaning doorknobs, phones, toilet seats and anywhere else that you need to watch for germs.

Ingredients:

16 ounces of water

3 tablespoons liquid castile soap
30 drops pure tea tree oil

Instructions:

Mix all of the ingredients together in a clean spray bottle and label appropriately.

Natural Dishwasher Detergent

This soap will work very well in the automatic dishwasher. However, if you have hard water, you may need to add ½ cup of vinegar to your rinse aid compartment to prevent a film on your dishes. If you have soft water, this won't be a problem.

Ingredients:

18 ounces of liquid castile soap
1 cup water
1 tablespoon lemon juice

Instructions:

Mix all the ingredients together in a quart-sized jar or container with a tight-fitting lid.

To use, add ¼ cup to the detergent compartment of your dishwasher.

145

Homemade Liquid Dish Soap

If you prefer to wash dishes by hand, this liquid soap works very well and smells wonderful.

Ingredients:

> ½ cup liquid castile soap
> 20 drops tea tree oil (for antibacterial help)
> 1/8 cup water
> 10 drops of your favorite essential oil, such as lemon or orange

Instructions:

In a large container, mix all of the ingredients together until well-blended. Pour into a clean dish soap bottle or repurposed container to store.

Homemade All-Purpose Cleaner

This is a great all-around cleaner for countertops, bathrooms, mirrors, tables and anywhere else you would use an all-purpose cleaner.

Ingredients:

> 1 teaspoon Borax

½ teaspoon washing soda
1 teaspoon liquid castile soap
10 drops essential oil (try lavender,
lemon or grapefruit for a nice, clean
scent)
2 cups warm distilled water

Instructions:

In a clean spray bottle, combine the Borax and
washing soda and shake to blend the two
powders. Add the liquid castile soap and your
choice of essential oil, then pour in the warm
distilled water. Gently shake while holding a
paper towel or thumb over the top of the bottle
(do not apply the cap, as it will foam too much)
and then cap.

Streak-Free Glass Cleaner

Vinegar and newsprint have been a favorite
natural glass-cleaning duo for years and they
still work great, although they can leave streaks
on mirrors and windows. This recipe makes a
glass-cleaner that is surprisingly streak-free. It
does contain isopropyl (rubbing) alcohol, so only
use if you know you're not sensitive to it.

Ingredients:

1/4 cup white vinegar

1/4 cup isopropyl alcohol
1 Tablespoon cornstarch (the cornstarch is what prevents streaks)
2 cups water

Instructions:

Mix all of the ingredients together in a spray bottle and use with a microfiber cloth or even clean newspaper.

Homemade Personal Care Products

Some of the products we put on our bodies most often are the same ones that contain the source of our contact dermatitis. Fortunately, many of the most commonly problematic products can be easily made at home and with excellent results.

Homemade Tea Tree Shampoo

This shampoo smells wonderful and creates an excellent lather.

Ingredients:

¼ cup distilled water
¼ cup liquid castile soap
10 drops tea tree oil

½ teaspoon grapeseed oil or extra light olive oil

Instructions:

Mix all ingredients very well in a medium bowl or container. Pour into a repurposed shampoo bottle. This mixture is thinner than most shampoos, so a little will go a long way.

Moisturizing Shampoo

This recipe is especially good if you have dry or damaged hair.

¼ cup distilled water
¼ cup liquid Castile Soap - your favorite scent
¼ cup aloe vera gel
1 teaspoon glycerin (available at pharmacies)
¼ teaspoon jojoba oil (in your health food store)

Instructions:

Mix all ingredients together in a large bowl or container and pour into a repurposed shampoo bottle. Shake before using, as the oils may separate on sitting.

Homemade Hair Conditioner

This hair conditioner produces great results and you can add any favorite essential oils that you like. Be sure to use distilled water as tap water may encourage the oils to break down.

Ingredients:

> 1-¼ teaspoon guar gum (from your health food or gluten free supplier)
> 1 teaspoon jojoba oil
> 5-10 drops of your favorite essential oils
> 1 cup distilled water

Instructions:

Add the guar gum to a clean, empty shampoo or squeeze bottle. Add the jojoba oil and essential oils and shake well to mix. Add the water and shake again. Be sure to store with the cap closed to prevent breakdown, as the ingredients are perishable and this mixture will only last about two weeks.

Moisturizing Shave Cream

This recipe turns out a beautifully light and moisturizing shave cream that is actually very luxurious. It will last about one month in an airtight container.

Ingredients:

4 tablespoons solid Shea butter (health food stores)

3 tablespoons coconut oil (available in the grocery)

2 Tablespoons sweet almond oil

10-12 drops of your favorite essential oil if desired

Instructions:

Heat the Shea butter and coconut oil in a double boiler or in a small bowl over a pan of simmering water. Stir until melted.

Remove from the heat and add the almond oil and any essential oils you'd like. Stir well and then place the bowl in the refrigerator until cooled.

Using a hand mixer, whip the mixture until frothy and smooth and then divide among covered glass jars or plastic containers. Keep in the fridge until ready to use.

Easy Coconut Oil Lip Balm

Many lip balms contain ingredients that are known to cause contact dermatitis in some people. That's unfortunate if you're one of those women who uses lip balm throughout the day. However, this recipe is wonderfully simple and the end result is comparable to any expensive lip balm from the stores.

Ingredients:

> 1 cup grated beeswax (available in the candle supply section of hobby and craft stores)
> 3 tablespoons coconut oil
> 1 teaspoons vitamin E oil
> 2-3 drops tea tree oil

Use a double boiler or a metal boil over a simmering pan of water to melt the beeswax. Add the coconut oil and stir until well-blended. Remove from heat.

Add the Vitamin E and tea tree oils and stir until combined.

Carefully pour into empty lip tins (repurposed or purchased from Amazon or hobby shops) and allow it to cool and harden somewhat before placing the lids.

As you can see, there is any number of products that you can replicate naturally at home for a fraction of the cost of commercial products and with the security of knowing that the ingredients are safe for your skin.

There are plenty of online resources for recipes such as these and many more. Once you start making your own products, you may well start a new hobby, or even a new business!

Conclusion

Having contact dermatitis isn't pleasant and it can be disruptive, but it doesn't have to run your life.

Once you know what is causing your contact dermatitis (and you may find there is more than one cause) you can take steps to avoid it altogether or at least reduce your exposure.

You can also do quite a few things at home to relieve the pain, reduce symptoms and speed healing. Making some lifestyle and nutritional changes can also go a long way toward reducing symptoms and even avoiding flare-ups altogether.

Finally, there are alternative products for those that are causing your problems, though you may have to spend some time looking and they may be more expensive than commercial products. If you prefer, there are hundreds of personal and household products that can be made at home very simply, using safe ingredients and for far less money than their commercial counterparts.

No, contact dermatitis isn't fun and it isn't convenient, but it can be largely avoided and controlled so that it interferes with your life as little as possible.

Appendix A – Products to watch out for

The first order of business when faced with contact dermatitis is to identify the source of the problem.

Once you identify the chemical or substance causing the problem, you next need to know how to avoid it. This isn't always a simple matter. That substance may be found in hundreds of common products, not just the hand soap (for example) that you've been using.

There are thousands of chemicals and naturally-occurring substances that are known to cause either irritant or allergic contact dermatitis. It would be nearly impossible to include all of them in this book.

However, what we can do is to include a number of the most common offenders, as well as the names of products that include those substances on a website for our readers. While this list may not by any means be an exhaustive list, it may help you to avoid your problem substance once it's been identified.

If you haven't yet seen a doctor for your symptoms, the list may also help you figure out which chemical is causing your contact dermatitis, though it must be stressed that there is no substitute for medical diagnosis.

The website address is www.contactdermatitiscare.com.

Appendix B: Resources for Safer Alternative Products

While there are a number of companies offering household and personal products that contain fewer problem ingredients, it's important to conduct your own due diligence.

While products advertised as organic or all-natural may be less likely to contain your problem substances, this isn't always a guarantee, especially if your problem is in fact a naturally-occurring ingredient.

Always read the ingredient lists for any product to make sure that it doesn't contain anything to which you're sensitive.

That said, these companies and websites specialize in more natural, safer products for home and body. One or more of these may prove to be an excellent resource for you.

Better Life

http://www.cleanhappens.com/

This company, started by two concerned fathers, offers a wide variety of household cleaning products, including dish and laundry detergents.

Arbonne International

http://www.arbonne.com/international.asp

This company has a huge array of personal care products, including cosmetics. Also makes nutritional supplements that are free of many synthetic types of filler. Products are sold online and through independent distributors worldwide.

Vitacost

http://www.vitacost.com/

This company is a huge resource for eco-friendly and natural products, but do pay careful attention to ingredients lists, as not all products are 100% "natural." This is also a great resource for pure castile soap, Borax, essential oils and many of the other ingredients for making your own products.

Shop Organic

http://www.shoporganic.com/prod_detail_list/green_products

This company has a good selection of organic household and personal care products. Again, watch labels, as some common irritants are organic.

Lily's Garden Herbals

http://www.lilysgardenherbals.com/index.html

This organic farmer and herbalist offers everything from face creams to shampoo, glass cleaner to sachets.

Gaia Natural Cleaners

http://www.gaianaturalcleaners.com/

This company offers a small, but lovely, collection of household cleaners, all made with minimal ingredients.

EccoBella

http://www.eccobella.com/

This company specializes in organic cosmetics, toiletries, skin care and even perfumes. Do make sure to read ingredients carefully, as many organic ingredients and essential oils can cause contact dermatitis.

Mrs. Meyers

http://www.mrsmeyers.com/home.jsp

This company's products use minimal and simple ingredients and may offer you a good alternative laundry detergent, household cleaner or air freshener.

Dr. Bronner

http://www.drbronner.com/

The leading brand of pure castile soap, this company offers castile soap with or without a number of favorite fragrances.

SunSense

http://www.sunsense.com.au/

Some of those with contact dermatitis caused by commercial sunscreens have reported that SunSense provided a great alternative for them.

The Honest Company

https://www.honest.com/

Founded by actress/product safety activist Jessica Alba, this company offers more eco-and body-friendly products made with fewer chemicals. Everything from sunscreen to toothpaste to diapers is offered and you can even request a subscription shipment to be delivered each month.

Works Cited

Bourke J, Coulson I, English J. "Guidelines for care of contact dermatitis." *British Journal of Dermatology*, 2001: December 154;6:877.

"Corticosteroids - Oral." *MedicineNet.* March 2, 2005. http://www.medicinenet.com/corticosteroids-oral/page2.htm (accessed March 14, 2014).

Foti C1, Bonamonte D, Cassano N, Vena GA, Angelini G. "Photoallergic contact dermatitis." *Giornale italiano di dermatologia e venereologia*, 2009: Oct;144(5):515-25.

Gonsalo, M. *Photopatch testing.* Author's proof, Journal article, Praceta Mota Pinto, Portugal: University of Coimbra , 2010.

Hogan D, Ellston D. "Contact dermatitis." *MedScape.* August 2013. http://emedicine.medscape.com/article/1

049353-overview (accessed February 21, 2014).

Hughes TM, Stone NM. "Benzophenone 4: an emerging allergen in cosmetics and toiletries?" *Contact Dermatitis*, 2007: Mar;56(3):153-6.

Jacobs D, Gross M, Tapsell L. "Food synergy: an operational concept for understanding nutrition." *American Journal of Clinical Nutrition*, 2009: May 89:5;(15453-15485).

Katsarou A, Armenaka M, Vosynioti V, Lagogianni E, Kalogeromitros D, Katsambas A. "Tacrolimus ointment 0.1% in the treatment of allergic contact eyelid dermatitis." *Journal of the Euopean Academy of Dermatology and Venereology*, 2009: Apr;23(4):382-7.

Katsarou A, Makris M, Papagiannaki K, Lagogianni E, Tagka A, Kalogeromitros D. "Tacrolimus 0.1% vs mometasone furoate topical treatment in allergic contact hand eczema: a prospective randomized clinical study." *European Journal of Dermatology*, 2012: Mar-Apr;22(2):192-6.

Kerr A, Ferguson J. "Photocontact Dermatitis." *Photodermatology, Photoimmunology and Photomedicine*, 2010: Apr;26(2):56-65.

Khandpur 1, Sharma VK, Sumanth K. "Topical immunomodulators in dermatology." *Journal of Postgraduate Medicine*, 2004: Apr-Jun;50(2):131-9.

Lewis, V. "Calcineurin inhibitors." *NetDoctor.* November 7, 2011. http://www.netdoctor.co.uk/skin_hair/eczema_cytokine_inhibitors_003766.htm (accessed March 15, 2014).

Matsukura T, Tanaka H. "Applicability of zinc complex of L-carnosine for medical use." *Biochemistry (Moscow Supplement)*, 2000: Jul;65(7):817-23.

Racanelli V, Rehermann B. "The Liver as an Immunological Organ." *Hepatology*, January 2006: Volume 1.

Rodríguez E1, Valbuena MC, Rey M, Porras de Quintana L. "Causal agents of photoallergic contact dermatitis diagnosed in the national institute of dermatology of Colombia."

Photodermatogoy, Photoimmunology and Photomedicine, 2006: Aug;22(4):189-92.

Scholz RW, Graham KS, Gumpricht , Reddy CC. "Mechanisms of interaction of Vitamin E and glutathione in the protection against membrane lipid peroxidation." *Annals of the New York Academy of Sciences*, 1989: 570:514-517.

Taylor J, Amado A. "Contact Dermatitis and Related Conditions." *Cleveland Clinic Center for Continuing Education.* 2014. http://www.clevelandclinicmeded.com/me dicalpubs/diseasemanagement/dermatol ogy/contact-dermatitis-and-related-conditions/ (accessed March 31, 2014).

Vilma A, et al. "Partial Sleep Restriction Activates Immune Response-Related Gene Expression Pathways: Experimental and Epidemiological Studies in Humans." *PLoS ONE*, n.d.: 2013.

Lightning Source UK Ltd.
Milton Keynes UK
UKHW02f0811190918
329159UK00009B/181/P